WITHDRAWN

THE CRIMINALIZATION
OF MEDICINE

THE CRIMINALIZATION
OF MEDICINE

America's War on Doctors

RONALD T. LIBBY

The Praeger Series on Contemporary Health and Living
Julie Silver, Series Editor

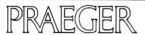

Westport, Connecticut
London

Library of Congress Cataloging-in-Publication Data

Libby, Ronald T.
The criminalization of medicine : America's war on doctors / Ronald T. Libby.
    p. ; cm. — (Praeger series on contemporary health and living,
    ISSN 1932–8079)
    Includes bibliographical references and index.
    ISBN-13: 978–0–313–34546–3 (alk. paper)
    1. Physicians–United States–Discipline.   2. Medical laws and legislation–United States.
3. Drug control–United States.   4. Medical care, Cost of–United States.
[DNLM: 1. United States. Drug Enforcement Administration.   2. Physicians–legislation &
jurisprudence–United States.   3. Ethics, Professional–United States.   4. Fraud–legislation &
jurisprudence–United States.   5. Prescriptions, Drug–United States.   6. Scapegoating–United
States.   7. Social Behavior–United States. W 32.5 AA1 L694c   2008]   I. Title.   II. Series.
    RA399.A3L48   2008
    362.17′2–dc22   2007039096

British Library Cataloguing in Publication Data is available.

Library of Congress Catalog Card Number: 2007039096
ISBN-13: 978–0–313–34546–3
ISSN: 1932–8079

First published in 2008

Praeger Publishers, 88 Post Road West, Westport, CT 06881
An imprint of Greenwood Publishing Group, Inc.
www.praeger.com

Printed in the United States of America

The paper used in this book complies with the
Permanent Paper Standard issued by the National
Information Standards Organization (Z39.48–1984).

10 9 8 7 6 5 4 3 2 1

To the memory of Dr. Benjamin Rutledge Moore and all physicians and their families whose lives have been shattered by unjust prosecution.

Contents

SERIES FOREWORD

Over the past hundred years, there have been incredible medical break-throughs that have prevented or cured illness in billions of people and helped many more improve their health while living with chronic conditions. A few of the most important twentieth-century discoveries include antibiotics, organ transplants, and vaccines. The twenty-first century has already heralded important new treatments including such things as a vaccine to prevent human papillomavirus from infecting and potentially leading to cervical cancer in women. Polio is on the verge of being eradicated worldwide, making it only the second infectious disease behind smallpox to ever be erased as a human health threat.

In this series, experts from many disciplines share with readers important and updated medical knowledge. All aspects of health are considered including subjects that are disease-specific and preventive medical care. Disseminating this information will help individuals to improve their health as well as researchers to determine where there are gaps in our current knowledge and policymakers to assess the most pressing needs in health care.

Series Editor Julie Silver, M.D.
Assistant Professor
Harvard Medical School
Department of Physical Medicine and Rehabiliation

PREFACE

The origins of this book are stories I was told by medical doctors who were close friends. I overheard discussions of fellow physicians who had been arrested and prosecuted for billing fraud and prescribing pain medication to patients. Their conversations were in hushed tones with a hint of fear in their voices. It was clear to me that they were confused and frightened by what was happening to doctors and worried that they could be next.

I was initially skeptical of these reports. Why would the government scapegoat the most humane and caring professional class in society? Perhaps this happened to marginalized groups in society but could it happen to an entire professional class—medical doctors? Even if the reported cases were true, perhaps they were isolated instances of corrupt doctors. On the other hand, if the cases represented a larger national trend, they could be just the tip of the iceberg? As incredulous as it initially sounded to me, the government could be targeting physicians for investigation and prosecution. If so, why would they do so? To answer these questions I set about investigating cases of doctors who were prosecuted for fraud and illegal prescribing to determine if they revealed a pattern of scapegoating. In other words, as a group, did these cases reveal the imprint of a national policy of targeting doctors for prosecution? Was there a pattern of egregious prosecutorial overreach or injustice? Did law enforcement have the same *modus operandi* in these cases? In order to investigate this proposition, I turned to major national medical associations for assistance. I asked state and national medical associations to announce my research to physicians throughout the country. This included the American Medical Association, the Florida Medical Association, California Medical Association, the Texas Medical Association, American Association of Surgeons and Physicians, and the Federation of Physicians and Dentists.

To my surprise, they all eagerly agreed to publicize my research in their newsletters. They did not regard my research hypothesis as ridiculous. It was not even necessary to explain in any detail the purpose of the research. Indeed, they talked to me confidentially and treated me as an insider with some hidden knowledge of their plight. In professional newsletters and Web sites, they announced that I wished to contact physicians who had been unjustly targeted by law enforcement agencies. My address and contact numbers were listed, and doctors were asked to relate their experiences to me. The announcement assured them of anonymity.

I had no idea what to expect from this. Indeed, the conventional wisdom is that doctors are busy professionals and that they had a built-in tendency to take whatever adversity life dealt them and suffer in silence. Others mentioned the proverb "Where there is smoke, there is fire." The government would not investigate a physician for criminal behavior they reasoned, unless there were solid grounds for doing so. Law enforcement agencies assured me that there were very few doctors who were actually investigated. To my great surprise, soon after the announcement of my research, I was inundated with hundreds of phone calls, e-mails, letters, and faxes from doctors all over the country. Indeed, more than one physician contacted me by phone at 2 A.M. in the morning confused by what was happening to him and desperately pleading for help.

What became immediately apparent to me was that physicians were extremely fearful of the government and wanted promises of anonymity. This presented me with a dilemma. If my research were to have any credibility, I would have to document the cases that were reported to me. However, physicians were frightened of having the government, and, as I later discovered, the insurance companies, find out that they had reported their cases to an outsider. One reason for their fear is that 95 percent of all those indicted for felonies plead guilty. As part of their plea agreement, they are forced to sign a document obligating them to keep their cases private. This meant that I was forced to rely upon the trials of physicians for the research that represent a tiny fraction of the total number of doctors who are indicted by the government.

After some reflection, I decided it was essential that I document the cases reported to me. In effect, I was forced to rely on cases that were already on the public record. However, even in these cases, physicians are reluctant to expose themselves and family members to further public humiliation by discussing their cases.

Indeed, the tragic case of Dr. Naren Jadeja, a young neonatologist who committed suicide rather than plead guilty to defrauding Medicaid, illustrates the extreme reluctance of physicians and their families to discuss their cases. Despite repeated attempts to persuade Dr. Jadeja's widow to provide documentation of the government's charges against her husband, she refused to grant permission for me to speak to her husband's attorney. Dr. Jadeja's professional colleagues even tried to persuade his wife to give me the documentation for his case. Several of his closest friends spoke to her, but the fear of disgracing the family was so great that she declined to provide any assistance.

Nevertheless, I did manage to persuade a number of physicians that if they were, indeed, innocent victims of abusive governmental action, it was imperative for them to tell their stories for the public record. This book represents an attempt to document their stories and to explain the government's draconian policy of harassing, and prosecuting physicians.

I owe my greatest debt of gratitude to my wife, Myriam C. Perez, M.D., who first brought the issue to my attention and introduced me to her circle of friends in medical practice. During the five years of research and writing of the book, she carefully guided me with the same professional skill and dedication she has always devoted to her patients. She read and reread every chapter of the book and offered advice at every stage of the project. Without her assistance, the book never would have been written.

I wish to thank Howard Fishman who wrote a series of articles for *The Psychiatric Times* exposing abuses of Medicare and Medicaid fraud investigators. I am grateful to Thomas M. Dawson and Nicholas W. Bartz, D.O., for their assistance with the cases of Dr. Benjamin Moore and Allan "Luke" Belden. Dawson read the entire manuscript. Kenneth Webster and Christie Nichols were helpful with the "Pinellas 14" case in Tampa, Florida. Patsy Vargo, M.D., was helpful in understanding her case in Montana. Monika Krizek Griffis, the daughter of Dr. George Krizek, provided the trial transcripts and discovery material for her father's case in Washington, DC. Lorraine Rutgard, the mother of Jeff Rutgard, M.D., was helpful with trial transcripts, discovery material, and background information necessary to understand her son's case in southern California. Jane Orient, M.D., the executive director of the American Association of Physicians and Surgeons (AAPS) based in Arizona was an important source of information and contacts for many of the cases discussed in the book and read the manuscript. Indeed, the AAPS is the only professional medical association that has sought to support physicians who have been unjustly targeted for prosecution.

Tom Bugle was important in providing background documentation for the case of Charles "Tom" Sell, D.D.S., in Missouri. Benjamin Moore was an important source of information about his case in North Carolina before his tragic suicide in 2002. Frank Fisher, M.D., provided background information for his case in northern California. James F. Graves, M.D., and his son Jimmy were helpful in assisting with the trial transcripts and background material in his case. William C. McLain, the public defender, and Russ Edgar, the Assistant State Attorney in Pensacola, Florida, provided insights into the prosecution of Dr. Graves.

Eli D. Stutsman provided assistance with the trial transcripts for the Comprehensive Care cases in South Carolina in 2002. Jeffrey Parker read the manuscript and offered valuable assistance with the legal analysis. I am grateful for the guidance and extraordinary editorial assistance from my agent James R. Cypher in the preparation of the book manuscript. Thanks to A. David Kline, the Director of the Blue Cross and Blue Shield Florida Center for Ethics, Public Policy, and Professions at the University of North Florida for giving me released time from teaching to complete the book. As always, my brilliant daughters, Erin K. Jenne and Kathleen E. Libby, provided inspiration for the book.

1

INTRODUCTION

The government has promised virtually unlimited health care to senior citizens.[1] According to the comptroller general of the United States, the health care system is not only unsustainable but if it is not reformed, it could bankrupt America.[2] The president and leaders of both political parties in Congress agree with this dire prediction, however, they have taken the easier course and have avoided making tough decisions to deal with the crisis.[3]

The government has also failed to win the war on drugs. For example, despite spending $600 million a year in Colombia since 2000 to eradicate cocaine production and end drug trafficking, there is no shortage of illegal cocaine in the United States. Congressional Democrats as well as Republicans have criticized failed drug war programs. In 2005, conservative antitax groups urged Congress to eliminate six failed drug war programs to save money in the wake of Hurricane Katrina. In 2006, the Republican Study Committee, a Congressional caucus of more than 100 conservative members, recommended the elimination of the High Intensity Drug Trafficking Areas program (HIDTA), the National Youth Anti-Drug Media Campaign Drug Initiative, Plan Colombia, and student drug testing grants to schools.[4]

SCAPEGOATING DOCTORS

Instead of addressing the underlying problems, politicians have employed a well-worn tradition of using scapegoats to blame the out-of-control costs of health care and the failure to win the war on drugs.[5] Doctors, among others, have been demonized for these twin evils.

The government's position is that there are adequate budgetary resources to fully fund Medicare and Medicaid and the only real threat to the health care system is fraud and waste perpetrated by doctors and other health professionals. Likewise, according to the government, a handful of greedy doctors are responsible for creating a new drug epidemic sweeping the country—prescription painkillers addicting patients and causing overdose deaths and injuries.[6] Thus doctors are held responsible for fraud and the distribution of dangerous narcotics for profit.

Medical doctors have come under the scrutiny of law enforcement agencies for civil and criminal investigation of felonies and they have been sent to jail for minor infractions such as bookkeeping errors and for prescribing pain medications to relieve patients' chronic pain.

THE WAR ON MEDICAL FRAUD

There is a widespread belief that huge sums of money have been defrauded from the country's $2.4 trillion annual health care spending and that the government has failed to stop it. Malcolm Sparrow, a former detective chief inspector with the British police and expert on American health fraud, claims that as much as $500 billion dollars is stolen from health care each year.[7] Sparrow believes that health fraud is massive, invisible, and uncontrolled. The National Health Care Anti-Fraud Association (NHCAA), comprised of 90 antifraud units in health insurance companies, federal, and state law enforcement agencies, echoes this theme. The NHCAA claims that most fraud is committed by physicians and other health professionals.

The public shares this perception of the country's plundered health care system. A poll commissioned by the American Association of Retired Persons (AARP) in 1998, for example, involving 2,000 respondents between the ages of 18 and 65 plus, confirms this belief.[8] The poll revealed that 83 percent felt health fraud was widespread, 72 percent thought that Medicare would become bankrupt because of fraud, and 76 percent believed that their personal health care is threatened by fraud. A recent opinion survey of 1,000 carried out by PricewaterhouseCoopers Health Research Institute in October 2006 revealed that 90 percent of respondents said that greed was causing rising health care costs. They ranked greed above all other factors including medical malpractice, the uninsured and administrative costs.[9]

The government has tapped this fear by creating a vast law enforcement bureaucracy to eradicate health fraud. Nevertheless, the public believes that investigations and prosecutions have not eliminated health fraud. Indeed, in 1997, the government tapped this pervasive public fear by creating toll-free telephone hotlines to report health care fraud. Thousands of reports of alleged health fraud are made on the hotline every month.

Targeting physicians as the principal source of health fraud and corruption is misdirected, however. Doctors' services constitute less than 24 percent of the cost of total health services.[10] Furthermore, for the last 10 years, their income has declined. Table 1.1 shows the decline in doctors' net income from 1996 to 2005.

This is in marked contrast with the huge salaries and profits enjoyed by the large health insurance companies. In 2005, William McGuire, the CEO of United Health Group, received over $8 million, Larry Glasscock, the CEO of WellPoint, Inc., received compensation of $5.2 million, Raymond McCaskey,

Table 1.1
Physicians' Median Net Earnings (in Thousands of Dollars), 1996–2005

Change since	1996	1998	2000	2003	2005	1996(%)
Family physicians	$125	$138	$130	$149	$150	−9.0
General practice	$105	$107	$ 90	$120	$150	+1.1
General surgeons	$185	$190	$200	$235	$233[a]	+1.0
Internists	$126	$142	$127	$150	$157	−9.4
Ob/gyns	$207	$196	$193	$208	$210	−7.7
Orthopedic surgeons	$258	$273	$277	$368	$300[a]	−9.6
Pediatricians	$129	$129	$131	$140	$150	−8.8
Increase in consumer price index						24.5%

Note: [a]2004 data. The CPI increase from 1996 to 2004 was 17.4%.
Source: Medical Economics Continuing Survey and the U.S. Bureau of Labor Statistics. Medical Economics Archive, Survey Report, "Earnings: Time to Call A Code Blue?" September 17, 2001, p. 4; "Exclusive Survey, Earnings: Primary Care Tries to Hang On," September 17, 2004; "Compare Your Earnings with Those of Colleagues in Your Specialty and Others. The News for Primary Care Physicians Is a Bit Better," October 20, 2006. U.S. Department of Labor, Bureau of Labor Statistics, Consumer Price Index, February 21, 2007.

the CEO of Health Care Service, Corporation received $6 million, and John Rowe, the Executive Chair of Aetna, Inc., was paid more than $3.1 million.[11] In 2005, the top five health insurance companies—United Health Group, Wellpoint, Aetna, Cigna, and Humana—declared profits totaling more than $9.3 billion while an estimated 46 million people did not have health insurance and drug prices and hospital stays were too expensive for many people to afford.[12]

In 2006, the top 10 U.S. health insurance companies had total market share of 53.5 percent and insured over 114 million patients (see Table 1.2). Insurance companies hired more than 500,000 physicians to deliver medical care to their insured members. That is about two-thirds of the estimated 800,000 practicing physicians in the country.

This has given these companies enormous economic bargaining power over doctors. It enables them to dictate the payments made to physicians and the services they can provide. If doctors do not sign the contracts with the companies, they automatically lose patients who are insured by the companies and risk being run out of business.

A consequence of the government's campaign against health fraud is that countless innocent physicians throughout the country have had their careers and lives destroyed. While the government acknowledges that more than 99 percent of physicians are honest, doctors have been indicted and prosecuted for murder, manslaughter, fraud, lying, rape, money laundering, racketeering, kickback schemes, mail fraud, and obstruction of justice.

Table 1.2
National Enrollment and Market Share for Top 10 U.S. Managed Care Organizations

Managed Care Organization	Enrollment[a]	Market Share[b] (%)
WellPoint, Inc.	27,236,851	13.21
United Health Group, Inc.	21,684,629	10.51
Aetna, Inc.	14,172,723	6.87
Health Care Service Corp.	12,262,905	5.95
CIGNA HealthCare, Inc.	9,064,024	4.40
Kaiser Permanente	8,825,581	4.28
Humana, Inc.	7,699,106	3.73
Blue Cross Blue Shield of Michigan	4,937,591	2.39
Highmark, Inc.	4,739,178	2.30
HIP Health Plan of New York	4,285,194	2.08
Total	*114,909,791*	*53.52*

Note: [a]Includes enrollment in HMOs, PPOs, POS, Medicaid and FFS-managed medical plans, for companies that offer fully insured managed care products; does not include specialty benefit enrollment. Enrollment as of fourth quarter 2006.
[b]Total national enrollment as a percentage of total national managed care enrollment as calculated by Atlantic Information Services, Inc.
Source: AIS's Directory of Health Plans: 2007. Reprinted with permission from Atlantic Information Services, Inc. 2007. Visit www.AISHealth.com for more information.

In contemporary America, it is a crime for a doctor to make a mistake when filling out a billing form for a health insurance company or Medicare and Medicaid for reimbursement. Furthermore, physicians are regularly convicted of violating rules and regulations that were adopted years after the alleged crime occurred.

The government has created a huge antifraud bureaucracy to investigate and prosecute doctors for the commission of felonies. Physicians have been tried and given longer prison sentences than convicted murderers; many have lost their practices, their licenses to practice medicine, their homes, their savings, and everything they own. Some have even committed suicide rather than face the public humiliation of being treated as criminals.

For example, Dr. Jeffrey Rutgard, a prominent San Diego ophthalmologist, was given an 11-year prison sentence, and his family's entire savings were seized for billing the government for "unnecessary" patient services in the amount of $64,000. Dr. Naren Jadeja, a young neonatologist in Bradenton, Florida, with a wife and three young children, committed suicide in 2000, just before he was to appear in court to plead guilty to a felony for charging the government for Medicaid services that were allegedly billed incorrectly or never provided.

There are hundreds of cases of huge fines, indictments, and imprisonment of physicians. There are numerous cases where, on the advice of their attorneys, doctors simply plead guilty to a single felony. The reason for this is that their attorneys tell them the only way to keep their homes and assets and protect their families from the humiliation of a trial, which they would probably lose in any case, is to accept the government's offer to plead guilty to a single felony count. As a result, many doctors have lost their licenses to practice medicine and paid huge fines simply to avoid the harsh publicity of a trial and bankruptcy due to the staggering costs of legal defense and the public humiliation to their families. Many physicians have unjustly been sent to prison.

Law enforcement agencies also employ extreme measures when investigating, indicting, and prosecuting physicians. They use the same tactics that are used against violent criminals, such as the Russian mafia and drug cartels. For example, in 1992, Dr. Rutgard's home and office were simultaneously invaded by federal agents with guns drawn at 6:00 A.M. Rutgard was ordered to awaken his wife and four children, ages one through five, and bring them into one room of the house where they could be guarded by one of the armed agents. The other agents proceeded to search the home and office. They collected 20,000 patient records and other documents, packed them in boxes, and removed them. To this day, the Rutgard's children are terrified by this experience.

Dr. Danny R. Westmoreland of Mason, West Virginia, had a similar experience. On June 23, 1995, Westmoreland's home, where he also has his office, was invaded by armed state and federal agents. The agents forced their way into his office with guns drawn and ordered the 15 to 20 patients in the waiting room to stand against the wall. This included his nine-year-old son who happened to be in the room at the time.

The case of Dr. Nass Ordoubadi of King County, Washington, also illustrates the extreme measures the government is prepared to go in investigating physicians. During the first week of May 1997, FBI agents visited four of Dr. Ordoubadi's clinics, posing as patients with make-believe complaints. They offered the receptionists fake identification and insurance cards. The agents tape-recorded their conversations with nurses and doctors at the clinics. When the FBI interrogated the clinic staff about fraudulent billing practices, Dr. Ordoubadi's personal finances quickly became the focus of their investigation. They asked questions such as "Does the doctor have a yacht? Does Dr. Ordoubadi have a vacation home in Europe? And where and how often does he travel overseas?"

They even coached Ordoubadi's physician assistant and partner in the practice to call the doctor during the late evening on May 13, 1997, to ask if the clinic was involved in any illegal billing. FBI agents were in the assistant's house secretly recording the entire conversation. Dr. Ordoubadi and his attorneys did not discover the secret wiretapping by the FBI until three years later.

DOCTORS AS SCAPEGOATS IN KICKBACK CONSPIRACIES

In addition to conducting commando-style armed invasions of physicians' homes and offices and terrifying their families and patients, the government has arrested and handcuffed physicians in front of their patients, used FBI surveillance and wiring as evidence against them, used disgruntled employees to testify against doctors, and intimidated patients into testifying against their physicians.

For example, in 1999, in Tampa, Florida, five independent family practice physicians received phone calls from the local U.S. Marshal's office ordering them to surrender by 1 P.M., or a bench warrant would be issued for their arrest and they would become fugitives. The doctors were handcuffed and chained by their ankles and brought before the judge. They were informed that they were guilty of a "conspiracy" to defraud the U.S. government despite the fact that they did not know one another.

The real culprits in the kickback conspiracy, the owners and manager of a medical laboratory who fraudulently billed the government for tests not performed, testified against the physicians. In exchange for their testimony, they were not only not indicted, but were allowed to keep all of the money they had defrauded the government and suffered no penalties except to be placed on probation.

SCAPEGOATING DOCTORS IN THE WAR ON DRUGS

Instead of addressing the issue of the failed war on illegal narcotics, political leaders have taken the easier course and declared that prescription opiates or narcotics is a greater threat to society than dangerous illegal drugs such as cocaine and heroin.[13]

Dr. Fritz Metellus, a Florida physician, was sentenced to 25 years in prison for allegedly trafficking in narcotics by prescribing pain medication to undercover deputy sheriffs posing as patients who claimed to be suffering excruciating intractable pain. Dr. Robert Weitzel, a Utah psychiatrist, was tried twice in 2000 and 2002, for allegedly murdering five terminally ill patients, ranging from 72 to 94 years of age, who were under his care in a terminal care ward of a nursing home.

In the chapters that follow, we shall examine cases of doctors who have fallen victim to the government's war on medical fraud, kickbacks, and drug diversion.

2

DECLINE IN THE STATUS OF DOCTORS: THE TRAGIC CASE OF DR. BENJAMIN MOORE

To understand why the government has targeted the medical profession for prosecution, it is necessary to understand the decline in the once-exalted status of physicians in America. In a 1959 book written by Allen Moore, M.D., we gain insight into the once-revered status of doctors in society. Dr. Moore was trained as a physician at the University of North Carolina (UNC). After his internship, he went to Doylestown, Bucks County, Pennsylvania, where he opened a practice. He was a personal friend and physician of the famous novelist James A. Michener, who grew up in Doylestown. Michener wrote these glowing words of admiration about Dr. Moore in the foreword to his book.

> Dr. Moore was on just about every significant committee and board in town. He helped lead the social life of our town and he could always be relied upon to take care of the people who simply had no money to pay. He lives on among us as the perfect example of a man who contributed mightily to the town in which he earned his living.[1]

Dr. Moore described another physician by the name of Dr. Dave Tayloe of Washington, North Carolina, in equally glowing terms.

> Dr. Dave was a physician of the old school. He was a combination of an old-fashioned doctor and a burning desire to pursue his medical training, with an intelligent grasp of anything new. He was your friend in health and your tower of strength in times of distress.[2]

Dr. Moore made two other notable observations in the book that help us appreciate the elevated social status of physicians at the time. The first is an event that occurred when he was a young physician working in the emergency room of a hospital in Philadelphia. A patient staggered into the emergency room in a highly agitated state, faking a seizure. Fearing that the patient might be having a heart attack, Dr. Moore ordered the nurse to administer a standard treatment of injecting the patient with morphine and atropine. The next day, while walking down the hospital corridor with the chief of surgery, Dr. Moore said that he was tricked into giving morphine to a narcotics addict. The chief of surgery replied that he had been practicing medicine for 35 years and "those fellows fool me every day."[3]

The other observation has to do with the importance and status of pharmacists. Dr. Moore referred to the town pharmacist as "a vital man in the community." No one ever hesitated to call on "doc." Moore elaborated by saying that the pharmacist "takes his place among the professional immortals."

> He gave us sound advice that was invaluable. He referred unsuspecting patients to us and told everyone that "Doc is a real good doctor, and he will take care of you."[4]

Almost 40 years later, Dr. Benjamin Moore, a physician and the grandson of Dr. Allen Moore, had an entirely different experience. His experience reveals the dramatic decline in the societal status of physicians.

Dr. Benjamin Moore was inspired by his grandfather to become a physician. In fact, he idolized his grandfather and shared his book with me. Dr. Moore was trained in neurology and pain management at his grandfather's *alma mater*, the University of North Carolina Hospitals at Chapel Hill. Moore had excellent credentials and outstanding recommendations from his employers throughout his seven-year practice history as a *locum tenens* or short-term physician.

As with most *locum tenens* doctors, Dr. Moore was forced to move in search of short-term employment while looking for a permanent position. As is the case with most new doctors, Dr. Moore had to repay large medical school loans. He had a short-term position in Laguna Beach, California, but once his contract ended, he could not find employment in California and thus was forced to leave the state in search of work.

He found a short-term position at the Onslow Memorial Hospital clinic in North Carolina. However, soon after he arrived, the hospital sold the clinic, and he was once again out of a job. Med-Pro, a *locum tenens* employment agency for physicians, found Dr. Moore another position in at the Comprehensive Care & Pain Management Center (hereafter termed Woodward's clinic), a chronic pain clinic, in Myrtle Beach, South Carolina. Med-Pro assured him that the owner and operator of the clinic, Dr. David M. Woodward, had a good reputation.[5]

Before he started working in May 2000 at Woodward's chronic pain clinic, Dr. Moore went to extraordinary lengths to ensure that he meticulously followed standard pain management guidelines as outlined by the Federation of State Medical Boards and the South Carolina Board of Medical Examiners and approved by the Drug Enforcement Agency.[6] Dr. Moore also carefully examined the American Pain Society's *Journal of the American Pain Association* and in particular articles on "opiate use for non-malignant pain." Dr. Moore contacted his *alma mater* at UNC and was reassured by his medical school professors that as long as he followed the state medical board's pain management guidelines, there would be no adverse repercussions.

DEA INVESTIGATION AND HARASSMENT

On June 13, 2000, just 18 days after Dr. Moore started working at Dr. Woodward's clinic, the U.S. Drug Enforcement Agency (DEA) raided it. A large contingent of DEA agents arrived at the clinic at 7:30 A.M. with guns drawn and brandished in front of the staff's children. They seized patient files, interrogated and intimated the staff, doctors, and patients. They told the office manager that she had better cooperate with them if she ever expected to see her children again.[7]

The agents asked the staff and physicians questions such as whether there were narcotics in the clinic, how many patients they saw daily (implying the clinic saw hundreds of patients a day simply to generate cash), whether they brought patients into a room *en masse* and wrote narcotics prescriptions for groups of patients without first examining them, whether the doctors had signed blank prescription forms, and whether Dr. Woodward asked patients to bring back their unused prescriptions (implying improper disposal of the drugs or possibly that Woodward himself was an addict).

When Dr. Moore arrived at the clinic at 9:00 A.M., the agents immediately ordered him to hand over his computer briefcase. A DEA agent searched Dr. Moore and his bag. The agent asked Moore for personal information such as his social security number. Moore refused to provide the number, believing that this was privileged information needed for tax purposes only. The agent responded that Dr. Moore had a "bad attitude" and said it may be necessary to mace and handcuff him. The agent also said, "Just because you're a doctor doesn't mean you're any better than anyone else!"[8] Dr. Moore instinctively thought that he was being harassed by the DEA precisely because he was a doctor.

Ben Moore subsequently informed the agent he had to go to the bathroom, and the agent followed him. Dr. Moore was then interrogated by two agents in a room without an attorney being present. He reluctantly agreed to this because he feared that if he refused, they would handcuff him, lead him away in a police van, and jail him with violent criminals and drug dealers. He later made the following observation about this humiliating experience:

> Why the rough tactics of intimidation and threat of restraint by the DEA on law-abiding, tax-paying peaceful citizens who have dedicated their lives to alleviating the pain and suffering of others? Last I heard, there haven't been a lot of reports of crazed gun-toting doctors shooting hapless federal agents or strangling Medicare or Medicaid auditors. Why does the DEA have to subject law-abiding employees in a doctor's office to tactics used in busting violent, paranoid, met-amphetamine users or suspected crack cocaine pushers surrounded by an arsenal of guns and assault rifles?[9]

After the DEA's raid of the pain clinic in June 2000, Moore panicked and contacted the DEA directly to determine what its guidelines were for prescribing pain medication. Of particular concern to Dr. Moore was a powerful synthetic painkiller called OxyContin. It is a narcotic painkiller comparable to codeine and morphine, which collectively are known as opioids. OxyContin was the only long-term pain medication he prescribed at the clinic.

OxyContin was an instant hit with physicians and pain patients soon after it was introduced in December 1995. The sale of OxyContin rose from zero in 1995 to 6.5 million prescriptions in 2000. It was the eighteenth best-selling drug in the country and the number one opioid painkiller.

Dr. Moore prescribed the drug because it was hailed by the manufacturer, Purdue Pharma of Stamford, Connecticut, as a breakthrough in the battle against long-term pain, and it was approved as safe for use by the Food and Drug Administration. The chief advantage OxyContin had was that it was a time-release pill that would give patients relief for up to 12 hours. Before OxyContin, it took between 496 and 992 short-acting pain pills per month every four to six hours to treat acute pain.

By contrast, a pain patient had to take only 60 OxyContin pills per month.[10] Physicians are reluctant to prescribe hundreds of opioid pain pills per patient every month. Indeed, the sheer volume of pain prescriptions written by doctors attracts the attention of the DEA and automatically sets in motion an investigation of physicians for possible illegal drug use.

Dr. Moore asked the local DEA "diverson control" officer, Linda Traube, if she thought he was prescribing OxyContin according to DEA guidelines. However, instead of answering Dr. Moore's question, Traube accused him of falsifying patients' records and said that he had now become a DEA target.[11] Moore took this to mean that since he had gone public by writing to members of Congress about the DEA's raid, he himself had become a target of investigation.

Ben Moore became particularly alarmed at Traube's response to his question about prescribing OxyContin. She said that only terminal cancer patients should be prescribed that medication. This set off alarm bells because up to 90 percent of OxyContin prescriptions are for noncancer pain patients.

This would exclude patients suffering from severe arthritis, back disorders, bone ulcers, and other illnesses. Indeed, the National Foundation for the Treatment of Pain estimates that 34 million people annually suffer from intractable pain that requires opioids for pain relief, with only about 5,000 physicians in the United States willing to prescribe opioids for these patients.[12] Since this is too few physicians to treat all pain patients, it means that family doctors have come under pressure to fill the gap.

Traube ended the conversation by advising Dr. Moore to seek an attorney's advice. Moore did just that and contacted an attorney, Joseph McCulloch, Jr. Dr. Moore told his attorney that the only long-acting opiate he prescribed was OxyContin because it was widely used by pain specialists who accepted the FDA and the drug manufacturer's claim that it was nonabusable and safe. Moore's attorney advised him that what he was doing was proper and consistent with the South Carolina Board of Medical Examiners.

NATIONAL CAMPAIGN AGAINST OXYCONTIN

Unbeknownst to Dr. Moore, however, the government had launched a political campaign against OxyContin in February 2001 after Dr. Moore joined Woodward's pain clinic. Hence, when Dr. Moore began prescribing OxyContin at the clinic, he was automatically targeted for investigation by the DEA. The DEA supervisor in the Columbia, South Carolina, office, Cheri Crowley, later revealed that Dr. Moore and five other physicians in Woodward's pain clinic had their DEA certificates suspended because they were inappropriately prescribing OxyContin.[13]

The DEA laid a political trap for Dr. Moore and other physicians who prescribed OxyContin to pain patients. They did this in response to a drug scare that became a media frenzy. OxyContin became the *cause celebre* in the government's war on drugs in early 2001. It was compared to the "crack cocaine epidemic" of the 1990s and was called "hillbilly heroin" or the poor man's heroin. It got this moniker because of its popularity in Appalachia and because it gave users a euphoric high when crushed and snorted. Law enforcement officials claimed that since illegal "street drugs" such as heroin and cocaine were not available in rural towns, addicts turned to OxyContin.

The political campaign against OxyContin began with "operation Oxyfest 2001," which was launched in Kentucky on February 6, 2001. Hundreds of Kentucky police fanned out in a five-county area, arresting 207 suspected drug dealers and users.[14] The media immediately picked up this story and quoted local officials who claimed that "abusers will kick a bag of cocaine aside to get to the Oxy."[15]

This resulted in a blizzard of media reports about an OxyContin epidemic sweeping the country in a rising tide of drug overdoses and a "narco-crime wave" of drugstore robberies searching for the killer drug. The so-called drug crisis was trumpeted to the nation in scores of newspapers and magazines, including *The New York Times, Time* magazine, *Newsweek*, and radio and TV programs such as "60 Minutes" and "20/20." Indeed, the U.S. government spends an estimated $25 million annually for antidrug advertising. Government advertising dollars were a powerful incentive for the media to create a media blitz in the war on OxyContin.[16]

Politicians quickly sought to capitalize on this publicity. For example, in March 2001, Virginia Attorney General Mark Earley convened an "Oxy-epidemic" summit meeting with top law enforcement officials from five states. The governor of Kentucky, Paul Patton, created an OxyContin task force for his state consisting of 15 law enforcement agencies.[17]

Not to be left out of the latest phase of the war on drugs, the U.S. Congress joined in the campaign against OxyContin. In a congressional appropriations bill considered in November 2001, the DEA was instructed to "redouble" its campaign to combat OxyContin abuse. The DEA's budget included money to help states track doctors and pharmacies, prescription of OxyContin and other narcotics. The authors of this provision, Frank Wolf (R-Va) and Shelley Moore Capito (R-W. Va), issued a statement that a strategy to combat Oxy-Contin is important because "the health of our families and communities is at stake."[18]

Evidence for the OxyContin Epidemic

Despite the national OxyContin drug scare and the political support for the campaign against it, there is reason to doubt that OxyContin constitutes a drug epidemic or, indeed, that it is even a major drug problem. There are several reasons for this. The first is that oxycodone is an opioid agent that has been used for about 60 years and is present in 58 different brand name medications, including OxyContin.

It is virtually impossible to determine in an autopsy whether OxyContin is the cause of death in a drug overdose. Traces of oxycodone may be found, but there is no way of knowing which is the formulation of oxycodone. Indeed, while OxyContin is the strongest oxycodone prescription, it accounts for only 25 percent of the total oxycodone consumed each year in the country.

Another reason to question whether there is an OxyContin epidemic is that despite a flood of media reports, there is no documentation of widespread OxyContin deaths. For example, law enforcement officials claimed that in the year 2000, the number of deaths in the country due to OxyContin ranged anywhere from 100 to 200. However, no medical examiner has been able to document more than a handful of deaths attributed primarily to the drug. For example, David W. Jones of the Kentucky's medical examiners' office was queried about a claim made by the U.S. Attorney for the Eastern District of Kentucky. The U.S. Attorney claimed that there were 59 OxyContin deaths in Kentucky in 2000. Jones said, "I have no idea where these people are getting their facts and figures."[19] He went on to say that there were only 27 "OxyContin-related" deaths in the entire state.

By contrast, there are reliable reports of about 17,000 Americans dying annually from the use of Advil and Aleve for the treatment of arthritis pain.[20] These moderate antiinflammatory pain drugs sometimes lead to internal bleeding, liver damage, ulcers, and death when taken frequently.

An additional reason to doubt the claim for an OxyContin epidemic is the fact that there has been no significant increase in the number of reported drug addicts in the country during the last 100 years. In 1914, for example, when narcotics such as cocaine was readily available in drug stores without a prescription, 1.3 percent of the population was addicted. In 1979, before the so-called war on drugs, the rate of addiction was 1.3 percent, and in 2001, the rate remained constant at about 1.3 percent of the population.[21] Thus, the rates of addiction in the country have remained constant regardless of the billions of dollars spent for the war on drugs, the growth in imprisoned drug dealers and addicts, and the widespread availability of narcotics in the country.

Indeed, the DEA has been unable to eliminate the illegal drug trade.[22] DEA officials acknowledge, for example, that most black-market narcotics come from crime syndicates in foreign countries where it is illegally manufactured. Therefore, instead of waging a losing battle, they have recently focused their attention upon controlling the legal prescription drug trade.

Unlike illegal drugs, the DEA can monitor all narcotic prescriptions by physicians. By staking out pain clinics and doctors, the DEA, with the help of local law enforcement agencies, is able to identify drug addicts and physicians who unknowingly prescribe narcotics to them. In effect, the DEA blames doctors for the criminal activity of addicts who obtain drugs from them under false pretenses. Doctors are also blamed for patients who overdose and die from misusing lawfully prescribed narcotics.

The effect of this has been to criminalize pain patients and their doctors and frighten physicians to refrain from treating pain patients.[23] The fear of DEA investigation runs so high that some doctors have gone so far as to put up signs in their offices saying "Do not ask me to refill pain medications" or "Don't ask for opioids."[24]

In the case of Dr. Moore, he vowed never to "prescribe medications for pain for anyone ever again, despite the need, because I now know that physicians are targets of regulatory agencies run amok, such as the DEA."[25] Ben Moore expressed the feelings of most physicians that they would rather be reprimanded by the medical board for undertreating pain than suffering the indignity of having their licenses suspended.

THE SOUTH CAROLINA WAR ON OXYCONTIN

South Carolina joined the war against OxyContin in June 2001, the same week that Dr. Woodward's clinic was closed and Dr. Moore and five other physicians in the clinic had their DEA licenses suspended. The state imposed the most rigorous restrictions in the country on OxyContin prescriptions. It required doctors to get permission from a state pharmacist before prescribing the drug. The state announced that only patients who have cancer, sickle cell anemia, or terminal illnesses would be eligible to receive OxyContin.

The law enforcement agencies investigating Dr. Moore were only too eager to accelerate their investigation of Woodward's clinic.[26] Based upon the Omnibus Crime Bill of 1984, all law enforcement agencies share the assets seized in combating drug trafficking. This means that law enforcement agencies can confiscate any cash, homes, boats, bank accounts, stock holdings, or anything tainted with drugs or drug money. It allows law enforcement agencies to take property without any charges being laid against physicians alleged to be drug traffickers. Police departments actually include money derived from drug seizures as part of their annual operating budgets.

The first step in the investigation was to survey 10 area pharmacies to obtain the number of doses of OxyContin and other opioids that physicians in the clinic prescribed. From this information, they constructed a list of physicians to investigate for illegally prescribing OxyContin.

The logic of the DEA's strategy was circular. Since the patients at Woodward's clinic were dependent upon narcotics, and since narcotics are addictive, pain patients are addicts. Applied to Dr. Moore, since he prescribed OxyContin to addicts, some of whom were criminals, drug dealers, or died from overdoses, he was a "danger to public health and safety."[27] The leap of logic from the criminal behavior of addicts to Ben Moore's guilt for unknowingly prescribing drugs to addicts is breathtaking. Not only is there no logical connection between the criminal behavior of addicts and physicians who have been tricked into prescribing drugs to them, but also do pain management physicians reject the concept of addiction in connection with pain patients altogether.

Physicians use the medical term "dependence" instead of the police term "addiction." Indeed, Dr. Moore argued that there is a huge difference between addiction and dependence. Pain patients are dependent upon narcotics for relief from pain that impairs their ability to be productive and enjoy life. This includes basic activities such a sleeping, doing chores at home, and walking and going to work.

Addicts, on the other hand, take drugs to get high and avoid life. Heroin addicts are lost to themselves, to their families, and to society. They cannot work and are likely to engage in criminal activity. On the other hand, pain patients get out of hospital, interact with their families, and go back to work when they are on opioids.

Furthermore, the medical evidence strongly indicates that patients who take opioids for the relief of pain are not dependent upon the drugs once they recover from the illness that produced the pain. For example, Henry Farkas, M.D., M.P.H. and medical director of the Northern Chesapeake Hospice, and a staff physician at Union Hospital, in Elkton, Maryland, said, "You will not make any patient an addict if you give them drugs to treat their pain."[28]

Addicts and Criminals Testify against Dr. Moore

The DEA accused Dr. Moore of willingly and recklessly prescribing narcotics to "doctor-shoppers," "addicts," and criminals without examining them.[29] The DEA's investigation report charged Dr. Moore with prescribing OxyContin to Mrs. Robin Anderson without a medical examination. Anderson claimed that she subsequently became an addict as a result of the prescription. This claim was made despite the fact that she admitted to buying the drug off the streets before seeing Dr. Moore.[30] Another pain patient, Charles Weatherford, who was arrested by the Darlington County Sheriff's office for burglary, testified that he fraudulently obtained OxyContin from Dr. Moore by claiming to have back pain. He said that he became addicted to the drug after crushing and injecting it.[31]

The DEA also charged Dr. Moore with unlawfully prescribing opioids based upon the testimony of Mr. Stanley Morgan, another fake pain patient. Morgan was arrested during an attempt to rob an Eckerd drug store in Hartsville, South Carolina. Morgan had previously obtained OxyContin fraudulently from Dr. Moore by claiming to have severe neck and back pain.

The DEA even used hearsay testimony of drug-dealing addicts who had never been treated by Dr. Moore to charge him with unlawfully prescribing narcotics. For example, James R. Woods, a drug dealer and addict, was arrested on May 31, 2001, for unlawful possession of OxyContin by the Darlington County Sheriff's Office and interrogated by the South Carolina Department of Health and Environmental Control, Bureau of Drug Control (DHEC). Woods testified that drug addicts and dealers around Hartsville, South Carolina, traveled to Woodward's clinic because they can "get what they want."[32] Woods also testified that 99 percent of the black-market OxyContin in the area came from Woodward's clinic.

Another DEA charge against Dr. Moore was that he had prescribed narcotics to doctor-shopping addicts who died from overdoses. For example, Gary Smith of Lancaster died from taking a deadly combination of methadone and benzodiazepines. Patricia Koks was found dead on July 1, 2000, due to multiple drug overdose. Timothy Scott Lunsford died on March 25, 2001, by overdosing on three drugs—oxycodone, alprazolam, and diazepam. And Richard Way was found dead on December 13, 2001, due to a drug overdose of hydrocodone and alprazolam. All of these patients ignored Dr. Moore's instructions and overdosed on a lethal cocktail of drugs.

Ben Moore went to great pains to try to weed out addicts, drug dealers, and drug abusers. He did this by routinely performing urine drug screens of patients and serum opiate levels to eliminate illegal drug abusers or multiple drug users. Indeed, in the last three months of his employment at the clinic, he terminated about 200 patients whom he felt were not legitimate pain patients. Nevertheless, the DEA charged Dr. Moore with violation of the Controlled Substances Act for "unlawful prescribing practices."[33] Dr. Moore tried to defend himself by saying that the DEA was blaming him for the criminal behavior of addicts who came to the clinic under false pretenses and for patients who died overdosing on drugs that were legally prescribed to them. Many of Dr. Moore's patients tried to avoid counseling, physical therapy, and testing. However, they were required to sign a treatment contract that made compulsory their full participation.

Indeed, during his one year at the clinic, Dr. Moore "discharged" about 300 patients who violated their contracts. Some had "track marks" on their arms (a sign of a heroin addiction), or they were suspected of being "doctor-shoppers." Ben Moore worked closely with the South Carolina Department of Health and Environmental Control (Bureau of Drug Control) to stop "doctor-shopping" and even helped prosecute violators.[34]

Ben Moore tried to rebut the DEA's accusations against him to no avail. For example, he said that Mrs. Robin Anderson was lying when she testified that Dr. Moore had not examined her. He said that he had, indeed, examined her and prescribed OxyContin because she claimed to have severe migraine headaches. He later discovered that she was a fraudulent pain patient and was abusing drugs by "shooting up" or injecting what she was prescribed. Stanley Morgan, who was arrested for attempting to rob a pharmacy with a knife, was not a legitimate pain patient. He was a "busted drug addict."

Likewise, James Woods was a drug dealer and addict who was arrested for unlawful possession of OxyContin. Woods' testimony that 99 percent of OxyContin on the streets came from Woodward's clinic was the opinion of an arrested drug dealer trying to get off drug charges by testifying against Dr. Moore. Charles Weatherford, who was arrested for burglary, also testified for the DEA against Dr. Moore for the same reason. Weatherford claimed that the OxyContin that Dr. Moore prescribed led to his addiction. However, he acknowledged that he had abused the OxyContin by crushing and injecting it. As to the deaths of pain patients due to overdoses of narcotics, Dr. Moore could say only that he could not be held responsible for patients' misuse of drugs.

The DEA also relied upon the opinions of pharmacists and the staff of drug rehabilitation centers to charge Dr. Moore of unlawfully prescribing OxyContin. In essence, there was a conspiracy of silence among medical professionals in the investigation of Dr. Moore. For example, in 1998, DEA Diversion Investigator Adam Roberson met with the pharmacists at 10 drug stores, plus Wal-Mart in Lancaster and Kershaw, South Carolina, to discuss Dr. Moore's prescribing practices. As a result of the investigation, all 10 pharmacies in the area stopped filling the opioid prescriptions of Dr. Moore and other physicians at the clinic. They took this action without notifying the physicians concerned and without any legal grounds for doing so. In other words, Dr. Moore and other physicians were being sanctioned by pharmacists because of the DEA investigation.

The pharmacists explained their action on the grounds that the patients were "strange out of town" people, they could not get verification of the patients from the clinic, they came in after business hours, they were not exhibiting sufficient pain to justify pain medication, and that they were known abusers or dealers of drugs.[35] The pharmacists also testified that Dr. Moore and other clinic doctors who were prescribing pain medication to these patients were not "legitimate physicians prescribing legitimate pain medications."[36] However, pharmacists were not medically qualified to make such judgments. They should not be the ones to decide who are legitimate patients and who are legitimate physicians. In effect, the DEA transformed pharmacists into law enforcement agents in their war on OxyContin.

Similarly, the staff at regional centers of drug treatment and detoxification centers testified that they had treated a number of OxyContin addicts who had received their medication from Dr. Moore and other physicians at Woodward's clinic. For example, Dr. Rene Lamm, a physician and addictionalogist at Counseling Associates of Georgetown, South Carolina, provided hearsay evidence that she saw patients who were addicted to OxyContin and that the patients said they "just go there (Woodward's clinic) and they'll give you whatever you need."[37]

Dr. Lamm said that "the community is scared" of Dr. Woodward, including pharmacists and other physicians. She said that Dr. Moore is the most ethical doctor at the clinic but stays there for the money.[38] Dr. Lamm did not have the professional courtesy to inform Dr. Moore or any other doctor at the clinic about the addicts she saw who fraudulently obtained narcotics from them. In other words, the DEA had also turned Dr. Moore's professional colleagues into agents of law enforcement.

The Destruction of Dr. Moore's Career

Without an opportunity for a hearing to defend himself, the DEA suspended Dr. Moore's certificate to prescribe narcotics to pain patients. This action is a career destroyer for physicians. Doctors whose DEA licenses are suspended are ruined forever. They can no longer be trusted by future employers and will be suspected of being guilty of the charges, whether ultimately exonerated of any wrongdoing or not. Hence, it effectively ends their medical careers. Dr. Moore was unemployed, was forced to vacate his apartment, return his rented furniture, and leave Myrtle Beach. He had no assets or salary and was forced to borrow $100,000 for an attorney to defend himself against further DEA legal action. He eventually moved back home to live with his mother and became deeply depressed. He was hospitalized for depression and in a fit of hopelessness, committed suicide by hanging himself in a tree one night in the backyard of his mother's home.

The contrast between the careers of Dr. Benjamin Moore and his grandfather, Dr. Allen Moore, could not be greater. Dr. Allen Moore was a highly respected member of the community whose medical judgment was not challenged by government authorities, pharmacists, or other physicians. By contrast, Dr. Ben Moore's medical judgment came under intense scrutiny and investigation by a score of law enforcement agencies second-guessing every one of his medical decisions.

His grandfather was tricked by an addict into giving him morphine without any legal repercussions. However, when Ben Moore made similar mistakes, he was charged with unlawfully prescribing narcotics and being a danger to public health and safety. Dr. Allen Moore trusted pharmacists to serve him and his patients. By contrast, pharmacists testified against Dr. Benjamin Moore and refused to fill his patients' prescriptions. Likewise, the DEA undermined physicians' professional ethics by using other doctors to testify against Dr. Moore. This contributed to the destruction of the career and life of an outstanding young physician. The most disturbing aspect of Dr. Moore's tragic ordeal, however, is that the government's case against him was based upon the testimony of addicts, drug dealers, and felons. This dramatically illustrates the fall from grace of the physician as an American icon.

3

MEDICAL MCCARTHYISM

The government has created an environment of fear among medical doctors comparable to the anti-Communist spy investigations of the 1940s and 1950s. The anti-Communist witch hunts during this period included Senator Joseph McCarthy's demagogic use of the Soviet and Chinese Communist menace to revive his fading electoral support and the hearings of the House Un-American Activities Committee (HUAC).

PHYSICIANS: ENEMIES OF THE STATE

The government has besieged medical doctors for allegedly being enemies of the nation's health. They are a key target in so far as they are the gatekeepers of the country's health care. Physicians authorize all health services, including hospitals, clinics, nursing homes, and medications. Therefore, medical doctors are the ideal scapegoats for the problems of health care in the country.

The Department of Justice (DOJ) has declared that fraudulent billing by physicians and other providers poses a significant "threat to the health and safety of countless Americans including the most vulnerable members of society."[1] With the passage of the Balanced Budget Act of 1997, Congress established a toll-free fraud and abuse "hotline" phone number for patients to report physicians for suspected fraud. This number is printed on every billing statement sent to patients. By mid-2000, the Office of Inspector General (OIG) reported receiving 48,000 calls a month on its fraud hotline.

Attorney General Janet Reno stated that "fighting healthcare fraud is one of this Administration's highest priorities."[2] California governor, Gray Davis, called anyone who defrauds health care "the scum of the earth" and vowed not to rest until "everyone is in prison."[3] In 2002, Sebastian Mallaby, the *Washington Post* editorial writer, declared that the country faces a national health scandal and "corrupt doctors" are the principal culprits.[4] At a Medicare compliance seminar in Oklahoma City in 2000, a lawyer who was formerly with the FBI and OIG of the Department of Health and Human Services (HHS) made the following statement.

> Physicians should make no mistake, the goal of the fraud and abuse hunters is to put each of you in jail. If that is not possible, they are there to retrieve monies.[5]

Even after the September 11, 2001, World Trade Center terrorist attack, the FBI regarded health fraud as the highest priority "white-collar" crime with a higher priority than violent street crime.[6]

The federal government created a national Health Care Fraud and Abuse Control Program (HCFACP) in 1996 under the joint command of the U.S. Attorney General and the secretary of the HHS. To coordinate the antifraud program, the government created a National Health Care Fraud and Abuse Task Force in 1999. It is chaired by the deputy Attorney General.

The task force brings together top law enforcement agencies at the federal, state, and local levels. It includes the HHS, National Association of Attorneys General, the National District Attorneys Association, the FBI, and the National Association of Medicaid Fraud Control Units.

There are regional health fraud task forces in each of the 93 U.S. Attorney's Offices (USAOs) that are headquartered in major cities throughout the country. There is an assistant U.S. Attorney in each office assigned to coordinate health fraud investigations. Typically, the USAO task forces meet monthly to consider cases of potential health fraud.

The health insurance companies that administer Medicare and Medicaid on behalf of the government also attend. At these meetings, the insurance companies present evidence of health fraud by physicians to the FBI, USAO, and state and local law enforcement agencies. This occurs without the knowledge of the doctors who are targets of fraud investigation.

The federal government lumps all law enforcement personnel together. They receive hazardous duty pay, can retire in 20 years, and have a very attractive retirement plan. All health fraud investigators carry guns. Despite some internal debate, officers want to have weapons. This is despite the fact that only one or two agents have ever been shot and not by physicians. Ronald D. Schwartz, the former deputy assistant inspector general of HHS asked the following question about the use of weapons.

> Does no one care about the traumatic and intimidating effect on the physicians, and their nurses, and their patients?[7]

Schwartz gave the following response.

> If you're the guy carrying the gun, you're unlikely to think in those terms. Besides feeling better about yourself and certainly more powerful, you would probably believe that because of the displayed gun, the person you're interviewing is more

likely to tell the truth. The law enforcement perspective holds that it doesn't make any difference whether the truth comes out voluntarily or at the point of a gun.[8]

In 2005, the USAOs had 1,689 health care fraud criminal cases pending involving 2,670 defendants. They received 935 new criminal cases involving 1,597 defendants. The USAOs filed criminal charges in 382 cases against 652 defendants and got 523 federal health care convictions. They also opened 778 new civil health care fraud cases and had 1,334 civil fraud cases pending.[9]

To investigate health fraud cases on behalf of the USAO, the FBI increased the number of agents assigned to health fraud from 112 in 1992 to 806 in 2005.[10] In 2006, the OIG had 85 offices in all 50 states, the District of Columbia, Puerto Rico, Guam, American Samoa, and the Virgin Islands.

PARALLELS WITH COMMUNIST WITCH HUNTS

There are parallels with the anti-Communist witch hunts of the 1940s and 1950s and the government's current war on physicians. Instead of targeting Communist subversives in Hollywood, trade unions, and universities, however, the government has singled out physicians and other health providers for jeopardizing the public's health and safety.

Comparable to the blacklist, the careers and lives of many innocent physicians have been ruined by government investigation, fines, and prosecution. They have lost their licenses to practice medicine, been bankrupted, ostracized by society, and many have been imprisoned. Even their own colleagues have testified against them on behalf of the government.

Parallel to Senator McCarthy's and HUAC's use of the media to destroy the reputations and careers of hundreds of alleged Communist subversives, the government uses the media to devastate the lives and careers of many innocent physicians. Ambitious prosecutors routinely alert the press of impending raids and arrests of physicians at their offices or homes. To get public credit, they arrange to have the press photograph doctors being arrested and clinics being closed. The arrest of high-profile defendants is a tried-and-true vehicle for advancing the political careers of prosecutors and securing positions for themselves in prestigious law firms.

The mainstream media are only too happy to publicize the investigation and arrest of high-profile, respected, and well-to-do physicians suspected of fraud. The spectacle of prominent and affluent doctors being brought down titillates the popular imagination.

The arrest of a major drug dealer seldom reaches the front pages of major newspapers or TV news. The arrest and prosecution of a prominent and successful physician, however, merits headline news. Most of the media would rather expose crooked doctors than defend innocent ones. It is extremely difficult for the media to speak out in defense of what the government definitively labels as fraud. Few reporters have a sufficient knowledge of medicine or medical law to question health fraud indictments. Therefore, many innocent medical doctors are tried in the media before any charges have been brought against them.

Analogous to the Communist witch hunts, the government relies heavily upon snitches for evidence of fraud committed by doctors. Snitches are close to physicians and therefore are trusted by them. This makes doctors vulnerable to acts of vengeance by jealous colleagues, disgruntled employees, personal enemies, unhappy patients, embittered ex-spouses, and family members who are social reformers.

According to Ronald D. Schwartz, the former deputy assistant inspector general of the HHS, there are two basic ways in which physicians are investigated. The first is that a nurse, bookkeeper, or colleague "rats" on a doctor to a fraud investigator. The second way is that physicians' computer billing records are inspected. They check to see if a doctor's billing pattern is higher or lower than other doctors in their specialty and location.

Schwartz points out that snitches are the most common reason for investigating doctors. He notes, however, that there are many reasons to turn in a doctor, and fraud investigators are not careful in evaluating the motivation of snitches. Schwartz elaborated this problem:

> I'm afraid that sometimes the investigators are not careful in assessing the informant's motivation. They're more likely to say: "Well, this person appears knowledgeable, so let's look at this doctor." I think that's how some of the bizarre, technical cases come about. The investigators are not technically trained. They know nothing about health or medicine. So, if they get such a call and find that the computer entries seem to confirm the allegations, they assume they've got a good case. And then, if they've invested a lot of time and energy, they may feel that they've got to get an outcome of a conviction or a money penalty.[11]

Incentives to Prosecute Doctors

In addition to snitches, investigations of medical doctors are instigated by so-called whistleblowers (called relators) who usually work in a doctor's office. Under the 1986 amendments to the False Claims Act 31 U.S.C. sec 3730(b), whistleblowers can file *qui tam* federal lawsuits entitling them to as much as 30 percent of the fine imposed upon a medical doctor convicted of fraud.

A billing clerk in a doctor's office who earns $10 an hour would be sorely tempted to testify against a doctor if he or she could get 20 percent of a $2 million fine. If a physician is convicted, the whistleblower receives the reward from the government even before the fine is paid.

The federal government pays out millions of dollars every year to whistleblowers in health fraud cases. For example, from October 1, 2000 to September 30, 2002, the federal government gave more than $311 million to whistleblowers. This money came from more than $3.7 billion the government collected in Medicare fines and fraud settlements with doctors and other providers.

Infringement of Doctors' Liberties

Similar to HUAC's violation of the Constitutional rights of witnesses, the civil liberties of physicians are frequently violated. The shield of civil liberties for citizens is the constitutional principle of *Mens Rea* or "no crime without intent." This concept requires the existence of a culpable mental state to find someone guilty of a crime. There must be evidence that a crime actually occurred, and the accused must be linked to that crime. No one should be prosecuted for an accidental or unintentional act. In other words, the government should not prosecute anyone solely on the basis of a theory or suspicion that a crime occurred.[12]

Medical doctors are denied this basic protection of the law. In the case of medical fraud, prosecutors usually do not even have evidence that a crime occurred until after the police seize physicians' records from their homes and offices.[13] After combing through thousands of patients' files for a year or more, the government typically selects a tiny sample of cases, usually fewer than 30, and charges a doctor with criminal or civil fraud. Conviction of fraud can result in huge fines and imprisonment.

Donald P. Zerendow, the chief of the Medicaid Fraud Control Unit in Massachusetts from 1978 to 1986, described what he termed the government's "extortion" of physicians on suspicion of fraud.

> Police don't walk into the home of a suspected bank robber and say, "Look, I think you stole $500,000 from the bank down the street. But if you agree to give back $300,000, I won't arrest you, charge you, and issue my standard 'Bank Robber Apprehended' press release." In some of the Medifraud cases, on the other hand, the investigator says to the physician, if you don't agree to this huge repayment which I'm demanding, based on my extrapolated estimate of what you've probably stolen, you'd better remember that I can bring criminal charges or a Civil Monetary Penalty lawsuit against you and let the press do you in. That clearly begins to resemble extortion.[14]

Unlike true fraud, however, that involves intentional misrepresentation, medical fraud can be unintentional or accidental. The government regularly brings charges against physicians for what they "should have known" rather than what they did know. This includes billing disputes, disagreements over what is "medically necessary," omissions on a patient's written chart or even illegibility of a doctor's handwriting. As far as the government is concerned, there is no such thing as an honest mistake by a doctor. Furthermore, the government does not even acknowledge the possibility that it could make a mistake in investigating and prosecuting physicians. Indeed, according to D. McCarty Thornton, chief counsel of the OIG in HHS, it is "simply not possible to convict a person for a mistake which is the product of an honest error."[15]

The government also refuses to acknowledge the possibility that innocent doctors have been investigated, fined, and tried for honest billing disputes. The combination of prosecutors' arrogance and power has resulted in many honest physicians being ensnared in the government's prosecutorial trap.

The government warns doctors that unless they fully document in writing the medical treatment given to every patient, they will be committing fraud. In other words, all bills submitted to insurance companies must be based upon what is written in patients' files (called charts). If doctors do not write down everything that they do for a patient, but bill for it, they could be fined $10,000 for each instance of "deliberate ignorance" and be subject to prosecution.

The government has broadened its definition of health fraud at a time that most "big-time" fraud in health care has been eliminated. Prosecutors are now increasingly forced to concentrate upon nit-picking technical interpretations of regulations to convict solo practitioners. Zerendow observes that health fraud investigations have changed dramatically from the late 1970s to the 1990s.[16] During the early 1970s and 1980s, investigators were dealing with doctors with clear criminal motivation. They investigated intricate scams that were cheating taxpayers out of huge amounts of money. This involved schemes such as medical labs that billed for tests that were never given, elaborate kickback schemes, and nursing home scandals that were widely publicized.

Since that time, however, there has been much less big-time fraud and more and more petty indictments involving clerical mistakes and misunderstandings of codes and documentation requirements. The reason is that most of the major fraud cases were effectively addressed during the early phase of the health fraud program.

Zerendow acknowledges that occasionally there are major fraud cases. These are the exceptions, however, and increasingly investigators go after small solo practitioners who are relatively easy to intimidate and overwhelm.

Federal "White Collar" Crimes

The growth in the regulatory powers of the federal bureaucracy is well known. When the Constitution was first ratified in 1791, there were only a few federal crimes such as treason, piracy, and counterfeiting. After the New Deal of the 1930s, an entirely new class of federal crimes was created to punish white-collar criminals. This includes the owners of companies that have accidentally damaged the environment and corporate CEOs who are blamed for the financial failure of their companies. Today, there are more than 3,000 statutory federal crimes and more than 10,000 regulatory crimes created by government bureaucrats.[17]

The new federal crimes differ from earlier crimes in at least four respects. First, the targets of prosecution are affluent upper-class professionals instead of lower-class street criminals. Second, the government no longer has to prove that the accused intended to commit a crime. Third, professionals are held criminally responsible for the actions of their underlings and associates. Fourth, white-collar criminals are prosecuted for *ex post facto* or retroactive laws. These are laws that did not exist at the time the crime was committed. Most environmental crimes are of this nature. For example, if a business is situated on or near a toxic waste site, the owners are criminally responsible for any environmental damage caused before they owned the firm.

Health fraud falls squarely into this category of new federal crimes. The government does not have to prove that a physician intended to commit a crime. Doctors are criminally liable for the billing mistakes of their office staff. Physicians are fined and prosecuted for fraud that was committed before the reported date of the fraud. In other words, fines and penalties are levied retroactively against doctors going back years before the date the fraud was detected.

The government uses what it calls "extrapolation" procedures to determine the extent of a physician's fine. For example, an investigator could say to a physician that "we have evidence that you over-billed by $12,000 over a six-month period." That represents $24,000 per year. "Since you have been participating in the program for the past six years, we expect you to write us a check for $144,000."[18]

Since 1996, the fines and prison sentences for medical doctors have dramatically increased. The amount of the fraud is now tripled plus $10,000 is added for each instance of overbilling. For example, $144,000 in damages now becomes $432,000 plus $10,000 for each instance of fraudulent billing. If there were 100 instances of fraudulent billing, the fine would be $1,000,000 plus $432,000 or $1.43 million.

The significance of increased fines is twofold. Antifraud prosecutors are now able to collect huge financial settlements from physicians and providers. It also means that federal mandatory sentencing guidelines (based upon the size of the fine) automatically dictate prison sentences. The bigger the fine, the longer the prison sentence. Prosecutors use the federal mandatory sentencing guidelines to intimidate doctors into pleading guilty to felonies and paying huge fines in exchange for a reduced prison sentence. As is the case with all federal crimes, 95 percent of criminal health fraud cases are settled by plea bargain and an even higher percentage of civil monetary cases are settled by plea bargain.

The federal government's malevolent attitude toward physicians and other providers is reflected in a statement made by a high-ranking official in the OIG of HHS.

> A doctor might say, "Really, those were all mistakes. I'm sorry." But we'll respond, "It did benefit you, so as far as we're concerned you're guilty of filing false claims. Now, let's sit down and talk about money." Then the doctor might say, "Well, I don't have that kind of money," to which we'll reply, "We're willing to accept your mortgage, and if you die, we'll also take your estate."[19]

Health fraud crimes are unique, however, even among federal crimes. The criminal laws that are used to convict physicians of fraud were created and interpreted by a private organization. Doctors are subject to criminal penalties based upon disputes over the billing codes that are owned and controlled by a private monopoly, the American Medical Association (AMA).

The AMA signed a secret contract with the government in 1983 to use its procedure (or CPT) codes with disease (or ICD-9) codes for use by doctors billing government health programs. In the 1990s, insurance companies adopted CPT codes for use by physicians billing the companies for the treatment of private patients. In effect, the government gave the AMA a monopoly over the codes all physicians must use to bill for their services.

The significance of the codes for the AMA is that about two-thirds of its $200 million annual revenues are derived from the sale of code books. The organization cannot support itself from membership dues alone. Indeed, only about 278 thousand or one-third of all physicians in the country are even members of the AMA.

All private physicians are forced to purchase the AMA's code books in order to bill for any medical service they provide. These books are continually updated, and doctors are forced to purchase these expensive books and spend a great deal of their time trying to understand them. This is like a patient tollgate on a freeway operated by the AMA. Every patient who is treated by a physician pays a user fee to the AMA. In 2002, there were 8,107 CPT codes that set the fees physicians were allowed to charge for medical services they provide to patients. Like ICD-9 codes, CPT codes are constantly changing. For example, the 2002 CPT codes had 700 changes from 2001.

The significance of the AMA's codes is that private rules and regulations are now used by the government to prosecute physicians. Any doctor who selects the wrong code or "mismatches" disease and treatment codes automatically commits a crime. Therefore, federal criminal laws have been created without Congressional approval and oversight and have been kept from the public.

In a twist of irony, the country's leading professional medical association, the AMA, has been seduced by the federal government's grant of a monopoly over doctor's billing codes. The association fears speaking out publicly in defense of innocent doctors who have been prosecuted for violating its codes. The loss of the AMA monopoly would immediately place it in financial crisis.

Voluminous and Incoherent Laws

In *The Federalist Papers* No. 62, James Madison warns us of the danger of laws that are so voluminous that they cannot be read and so incoherent that they cannot be understood. If laws are constantly changing so that no one knows what it is, or what it will be tomorrow, it is useless as a guideline for behavior. If it is no longer possible to distinguish between legal and illegal behavior, the law becomes capricious, unpredictable, and a threat to everyone.

Physicians are confronted with just such a conundrum. The laws and regulations governing medical procedures and billing are voluminous, ambiguous, complex, and are constantly changing. Medicare regulations alone are

110,000 pages long compared to 17,000 pages of IRS regulations. And there are thousands of procedure and billing codes that change continuously.

There are two sets of codes that physicians use for patient diagnosis and billing. The first is the International Classification of Disease (ninth revision) called ICD-9 codes. This is a list of 4,400 diseases with code numbers that physicians use to diagnose patients. It was originally developed by the World Health Organization (WHO) but is now managed and updated by the National Center for Health Statistics on behalf of the AMA. These codes do not cover all possible combinations of diseases and are, therefore, dependent upon a physician's subjective judgment. For example, disease code V62.4 is "social maladjustment" possibly due to "cultural deprivation," "political, religious or sex discrimination," "social isolation or persecution."

According to Fredric Steinberg, M.D., of Decatur, Georgia, this code defies medical diagnosis. What are the patient's complaints? What are the symptoms? What are the lab tests to rule out or confirm the diagnosis? What are the standards of care? And what is the reimbursement? Steinberg explains that not a day goes by that he cannot find an ICD-9 disease code to fit a patient's diagnosis. That means that he must use his best judgment to find a suitable code.

After finding a disease code (ICD-9) to diagnose an illness, a doctor must then match that code with a treatment code called Current Procedural Terminology (CPT) code. CPT codes are a list of more than 8,000 procedures and services provided by physicians to patients. Each CPT code has a fee that the doctor is allowed to charge. It is physicians' selection of CPT codes that is audited for health fraud. Indeed, auditors make a living second-guessing doctors' selection of the correct CPT code to use when billing for medical services given to patients. Auditors even receive bonuses for denying payment to doctors for using the wrong CPT code. This makes all physicians highly vulnerable to prosecution for fraud. Two hypothetical examples will illustrate the point.[20]

A 50-year-old white female comes to a doctor's office as a new patient, complaining she is gaining weight while dieting, is cold all the time, and her muscles ache. She has trouble staying awake at work, experiences fatigue, and her hair is thinning. The doctor does a complete examination of the woman and finds she is normal except that her skin is dry, hair is thin, and she appears sleepy. The doctor says, "I want you to have some blood tests and get your medical records from your previous doctor. I want you to return in one week with the records, and we will review the blood test results at that time." The doctor's diagnosis is that the women suffers from hypothyroidism (insufficient hormone production by the thyroid gland), which is a common disease for women her age. The doctor finds the ICD-9 code for hypothyroidism and bills the patient's insurance company for a CPT code of a new patient's initial office visit. The patient leaves the office and the bill is transmitted by computer that night to the insurance company.

After a week elapsed, the patient returns to see the doctor and get the blood results. The blood test show that the patient is normal and does not have hypothyroidism. The doctor had mistakenly diagnosed the patient based upon clinical impressions without, however, the blood test results.

The physician could be found guilty of fraud because he billed the insurance company for the wrong diagnosis. On the other hand, if the doctor had not made the diagnosis, the insurance company would not have paid for the blood tests necessary to confirm or rule out the diagnosis. Indeed, ordering tests for the purpose of excluding the possibility of a disease is itself fraudulent.

Another example of the impossibility of avoiding fraud as defined by the government is a patient who comes to see a doctor with a large, angry, black mole and a family history of melanoma (skin cancer). The doctor is immediately placed in a dilemma. There are two disease codes for this. One is for a benign growth, and the other is for a cancerous growth. The procedure code for removing a benign growth pays the physician $50, whereas the code for removing a cancerous growth pays $150.

The doctor cannot know which type of growth it is until a biopsy is performed and the lab results come back in about a week. If the doctor codes the growth as benign, submits the bill, and it turns out to be cancerous, he is guilty of fraud. Likewise, if the doctor codes the growth as cancerous and it turns out to be benign, he is also guilty of fraud because the disease code does not match the procedure code. This is truly a catch-22 situation against which there is no protection for physicians from arbitrary and capricious investigation and prosecution.

In both examples of the ambiguity surrounding doctors' coding and billing, all that is needed to initiate a fraud investigation is for a vengeful snitch or a whistleblower to report fraudulent billing to an investigator. This is a nightmare that all doctors live with daily in their medical practice. Criminal fraud charges can be brought against any physician or provider based upon minor technical violations such as coding errors or ambiguities of Medicare, Medicaid, and insurance regulations. Donald Zerendow explains the vulnerability of physicians to fraud investigators.

> Every misplaced file or "poorly documented" record represents a service that was not rendered; all recurrent treatment is "over utilization"; any procedure that cannot be easily pigeon-holed into an arbitrarily defined code is a source of "overpayment"; every clerical error in the physician's favor is "fraudulent billing"; and "exceeding computer parameters" is a flag of guilt.[21]

Howard Fishman, the senior editor of *The Psychiatric Times*, pointed out to a large audience of physicians that anyone of them can be a target of fraud investigation. He elaborated this theme.

> If you allow me two days to rummage through your medical records and billing files and to interview some of your patients, I guarantee that I can come up

with reasons to indict almost every one of you. And the charges will be identical to the charges that have been brought against any number of the victims I've interviewed.[22]

Incriminating Doctor's Notes

Prosecutors regularly use physicians' medical notes to investigate and try them for fraud. Samuel A. Nigro, M.D., argues that this is not only detrimental to the practice of medicine, but it is an exercise in futility and a waste of time.[23]

Physicians' notes were never intended for use in legal proceedings. Indeed, the very nature of doctors' patient records does not lend itself to legal proceedings. Nigro points out that physicians typically engage in a rapid succession of intense patient episodes. There are four stages of patient treatment. First, the doctor must establish trust with the patient; second, he must focus on the problem; third, he must arrive at a reasonable judgment; and fourth, he must implement treatment. All of this must be done within a matter of minutes. The doctor must clear his mind so that he can move on to the next patient.

Typically, physicians do this dozens of times a day and hundreds of times a week. To cope with this complex task, they hurriedly scribble notes on patients' charts and include a key word to trigger their memory at the next visit. Doctors' notes are written for the purpose of practicing medicine, not for use in court proceedings. Indeed, the idea that doctors' notes can form the basis of a court record is absurd. With tongue in cheek, Dr. Nigro says that if prosecutors want a complete and accurate transcript, a court reporter should be present at all doctors' visits. He also observes that if all medical records are opened for legal purposes, then the personal notes of judges and attorneys (called "work products") should also be opened to public scrutiny.

In court depositions, lawyers typically ask physicians in excruciating detail, line by line, what they meant by a particular notation in a patient's file written a year or more ago. With every word and phrase, the prosecutor reads their own interpretation into the record. If the doctor cannot recall exactly what was meant by every notation, it is used as evidence of fraud.

Ineptitude of Auditors

Another threat to physicians is that insurance auditors who review physicians' records for fraud are often not qualified to understand the treatment that doctors write on patients' files. Most auditors are not medically trained. Sometimes, licensed vocational nurses review physicians' records. They have only two years of training, however, and are not really qualified to review doctors' files.

That means that doctors' written comments on patients' charts (called "bullets") are frequently misunderstood. In other words, fraud investigators who lack medical training may unintentionally misconstrue evidence of overbilling.

Linda W. Wilson, M.D., of Culver City, California, notes that despite typing up three pages of notes per patient visit, her insurance claims were often denied by Transamerica, her Medicare carrier, on grounds of "lack of complexity and medical necessity." Her claims are always reviewed by nonmedical personnel, and they always result in nonpayment. Indeed, on the rare occasions that Dr. Wilson questions the auditors, she receives "reams of paper with jumbled-up paragraphs that make no medical sense."[24]

The case of John F. Kiraly III, M.D., illustrates incompetent insurance auditors imposing a fine upon an innocent physician. Dr. John F. Kiraly, a Lodi, California, cancer specialist, was audited by the National Heritage Insurance Company on behalf of Medicare. Heritage claimed that Dr. Kiraly had overcharged Medicare for patients' chemotherapy treatment. Heritage examined 2,694 billing claims submitted by Dr. Kiraly for 30 patients receiving weekly chemotherapy treatments during six months. After matching John Kiraly's billing records with the patients' charts, they could find only six instances where the charts did not justify the amount that was billed. They also found cases where Dr. Kiraly had undercharged Medicare but they were ignored.

Heritage calculated the amount of "overcharge" for the six bills, multiplied it times two (for the entire year) and then multiplied it times the number of bills submitted for all of Dr. Kiraly's chemotherapy patients during the previous five years. In other words, the government fined John Kiraly for suspicion of overcharging all of his chemotherapy patients without even looking at their records. This is not only a retroactive penalty, but the insurance company acted as Kiraly's judge and jury in imposing a heavy fine.

Heritage said that John Kiraly owed the government $57,975.93 and gave him 30 days to pay the fine or it would impose an addition penalty of an annual interest rate charge of 13.375 percent. Dr. Kiraly paid the fine but vowed to vindicate himself against the charges.

John Kiraly and his wife, Rena, who was his office manager and nurse, tried to persuade Heritage that they had not overbilled Medicare. Every effort to contact the insurance company to explain the billing dispute, however, was rebuffed.

After two and a half years, $10,000 in expenses and lost earnings from time away from the office, Dr. Kiraly finally succeeded in overturning the fine. He discovered that the company had misclassified his practice as a family practice rather than as a hematology and oncology practice. The auditors who reviewed his records were not qualified to audit oncology/hematology reports.

Despite Dr. Kiraly's pyrrhic victory, however, scores of physicians throughout the country are egregiously and arbitrarily fined by the government without a hearing or trial. Unlike Dr. Kiraly, most physicians are unwilling to challenge the government. They are fearful of retaliation. An insurance company can get revenge against a rebellious doctor by simply removing him from their list of approved physicians, or the government can deny physicians the right to treat Medicare and Medicaid patients. There is no trial or hearing, and these actions cannot be appealed.

This form of reprisal can mean the end of a doctor's practice. Even worse, if a doctor does not promptly pay the fine, the insurance company can turn the case over to law enforcement agencies for criminal prosecution. Hence, most physicians meekly pay the fine without question, or they quietly close their practices and go out of business.

Origins of the Antifraud Bureaucracy

Federal health fraud prosecution in the United States is relatively recent, dating from the late 1970s. After the passage of Medicare and Medicaid in 1965, the government was concerned about getting physicians to participate in the programs. Little thought was given to the possibility that doctors and other providers would defraud the government. A series of scandals during the 1970s, however, triggered a public outcry and changed the government's lack of concern about health fraud. The so-called FBI Labscam on the West Coast in which labs gave doctors kickbacks for referring patients and New York nursing home scandals in particular focused public attention upon health fraud.

The public questioned the failure of the government to combat fraud. This was acutely embarrassing to the federal department of Health, Education and Welfare (HEW) and to the Social Security's Bureau of Health Insurance, which oversaw Medicare. At the time, there were few, if any, federal health fraud investigators for either Medicare or Medicaid.

In 1975, Congress responded to the public outcry by creating an OIG in HEW—now the HHS. The inspector general's job was to eliminate fraud in government health programs. The inspector general (IG) was the chief law enforcement executive for the entire department. Congress also created a small Criminal Office of Investigations in HEW. Fraud investigation was soon expanded, and a large number of auditors were added to the staff.

The government's initial concern was with Medicare, but Medicaid fraud was soon added to the responsibilities of the IG. In 1978, Congress created Medicaid fraud units in the states and provided 90 percent of their funding for the first three years and thereafter provided 75 percent of funding. Control over their budgets gave the IG the authority to investigate Medicaid as well as Medicare fraud.

The federal health fraud bureaucracy underwent dramatic expansion in 1981. During the 1980 election, Reagan campaigned on a platform pledging to root out government fraud, waste, and abuse. One of Reagan's first actions as president-elect was to fire all 15 IGs in the government and replace them with "meaner junkyard dogs."

In place of the dismissed IG of HHS, Reagan appointed Richard P. Kusserow, a former FBI agent and Defense Department fraud investigator. In a June 1982 article in *The Washingtonian*, Kusserow was described as one of the five "junkyard dogs" who had an important role to play in Reagan's war on waste and fraud in federal programs.[25]

Donald Zerendow described the "junkyard dog" mentality in the following way.

> This meant that we were to be like growling, hungry animals who would show no mercy to perceived wrongdoers. This, of course, was intended to create an atmosphere of deterrence. But, in my opinion, it has instead resulted in an atmosphere of terror.[26]

Kusserow frequently made threatening statements to the press such as "I'm going to get you. We know who the cheaters are, and we're going to get you."[27] The antifraud bureaucracy had an overarching objective, however. That was to control the burgeoning costs of Medicare and Medicaid by discouraging physicians from treating patients. Jay Cutler, the special counsel and director of government relations of the American Psychiatric Association, made the following observation.

> If you treat patients, it costs the system money. While finding a physician guilty of fraud leads to criminal penalties, including monetary reimbursements and fines.[28]

The 10 Percent Myth

During Kusserow's tenure as IG of HHS from 1981 to 1992, he inaugurated a veritable reign of terror against physicians and other providers. Kusserow encouraged trivial and malicious prosecutions of doctors for alleged fraud of less than a hundred dollars. In his eagerness to demonstrate widespread health fraud, he routinely violated doctors' due process of the law in order to achieve high conviction rates and collect large fines.

Indeed, Kusserow was responsible for creating the myth that 10 percent of the government's health care expenditure is defrauded. In fact, to this day, politicians routinely cite this figure as the justification for spending billions of dollars on health fraud investigations and prosecutions.

According to Donald Zerendow, shortly after Kusserow became the IG in 1981, he pulled this figure out of thin air and presented it in an article published by HHS. Kusserow offered no evidence or documentation for the estimate.[29] Nevertheless, politicians accepted the 10 percent fraud estimate as factual.

Jane Orient, criticizes the myth by exposing the implications of such a claim. Ten percent of total government health care spending in 1998 was $100 billion or $100,000 million. If each thief managed to steal one million dollars annually, it would take 100,000 doctors to reach $100 billion. However, most doctors do not even gross a million dollars in revenue. There are only about 450,000 doctors in private practice. Therefore, if one doctor in 4.5 is guilty of fraud, it would mean that almost 25 percent of all private physicians would be massively defrauding the government.

Even the government denies this and acknowledges that more than 90 percent of all physicians are honest and ethical. Therefore, if the 10 percent estimate of fraud were correct, it contradicts the government's claim that they are only after a "few bad apples." A more reasonable assumption would be that most of the fraud is committed by large institutions or scams such as fraudulent laboratories or medical suppliers without the involvement of physicians.

Even in this scenario, however, there is no evidence to support the 10 percent myth. Indeed, as is the case with all mythology, it is not a hypothesis to be tested but rather a self-fulfilling prophecy for fraud investigators, requiring more and more investigations and prosecutions of physicians and providers.

According to Zerendow, the ability of the antifraud bureaucracy to exist depends upon two things. The first is its ability to convince Congress and state legislators that health fraud is rampant in the country in order to assure continued funding. The second is to produce good "statistics" on the numbers of health fraud convictions, exclusions of doctors and providers from Medicare and Medicaid, and collection of large fines and penalties.[30]

Kusserow's strong-arm tactics resulted in the "statistical" achievements necessary to secure continued support from Congress and state legislatures. For example, from 1985 to 1989, Kusserow reported to Congress that his office collected $29 billion in fraud settlements and fines and initiated about 5,800 successful prosecutions. For this achievement, Congress rewarded the IG's Office with a budget of $57.5 million in 1992.

The IG's Merit Pay/Bounty System

Kusserow created a tyrannical enforcement system for the prosecution and punishment of medical doctors and providers. He instituted a merit pay/bounty system that required all agents in the IG's office to meet conviction and monetary quotas in order to qualify for pay increases.

Kusserow repeatedly denied that the IG had conviction quotas. He was exposed, however, when U.S. District Court Judge Robert E. Coyle of Fresno, California, ordered Kusserow to discontinue the quota system. The case was brought by Kenneth Melashenko, M.D., in 1987, who appealed the IG's decision to exclude him from Medicare.

In 1990, Judge Coyle ruled that Dr. Melashenko's due process rights had been denied because of the IG's practice of awarding merit pay to agents for punishing physicians. In other words, fraud investigators in the IG's office had a financial interest in prosecuting medical doctors. This amounted to placing a bounty on the heads of physicians. As was the case with HUAC, the IG was acting as both judge and jury in destroying the reputations and careers of medical doctors.

The California Medical Association (CMA) entered the case on behalf of Dr. Melashenko and through a court order was able to confirm the IG's quota system. The CMA got hold of the personnel records of James Patton, the director of the IG's Division of Health Care Administrative Sanctions. He was the agent responsible for the decision to remove Dr. Melashenko from the Medicare program.

Patton's 1984–1985 personnel record revealed that he had to impose "10 percent more sanctions" than the previous year in order to qualify for a Level II merit pay increase. That would amount to 390 convictions and nine million dollars. In Patton's 1985–1986 personnel record, he had to have 430 convictions and collect $12 million in fines to receive a Level II merit pay increase. To receive Level III merit pay increases in both years, Patton had to exceed 10 percent of the number of successful convictions in dollar penalties.[31]

Kusserow created a system of rewards in the OIG in which in order to receive pay increases, auditors had to uncover "X" millions of dollars in fraud, investigators had to have "X" number of convictions of physicians and providers, "X" dollars of money penalties, and had to remove "X" number of doctors from Medicare and Medicaid programs.

Kusserow also set conviction quotas for state Medicaid fraud units. He did this by issuing directives on how each unit could spend its money. He also sent out special OIG teams every year to certify each state fraud unit.

In fact, Kusserow ranked state fraud units in terms of their "statistical" performance measured by the number of indictments, prosecutions, and size of fines they recovered. The units that had good statistics were called "preeminent" and ones that had bad statistics were "bottom" units. Implicit in this system was the assumption that fraud was randomly distributed throughout the country. Hence, it was assumed that the incidence of medical fraud was the same in New Mexico and Idaho as it was in New York or Illinois. States that failed to meet their quotas were suspended and threatened with termination. Nebraska and South Dakota were suspended, and others were threatened with suspension and termination.

Kusserow even warned fraud units not to reach administrative settlements with physicians and providers that allowed them to continue participating in Medicare and Medicaid programs. He wanted to ensure that fraud units had high conviction rates in order to convince Congress he was doing a good job.[32]

Kusserow's Reign of Terror

What statistics fail to reveal, however, is the wanton destruction of the lives and careers of many innocent physicians who have been prosecuted and fined. A few examples will illustrate the petty and vindictive nature of the OIG's prosecution under Kusserow.

One of Kusserow's most loyal lieutenants was George Yamamoto, the chief of the Hawaii Medicaid Fraud Control Unit. Under Yamamoto's direction, scores of physicians were prosecuted for fraud, some were jailed, and others left Hawaii. In one case, he prosecuted an optician who was convicted of a criminal felony for overbilling Medicaid by $7.75.

Fraud investigators prefer criminal prosecution of fraud, even for small amounts of money, to administrative hearings to resolve billing mistakes. The reason is that the prosecution of fraud serves a political purpose. Investigators must find fraud even if none exists in order to justify the federal funding they receive.

Yamamoto defended this criminal felony prosecution by saying fraud is a crime regardless of the amount. The American Civil Liberties Union testified against Yamamoto's "Gestapo tactics" of bursting into offices with guns and prosecuting physicians for small amounts of money. It condemned the government's use of "unchecked, unrestrained, and unlimited power which denies the due process rights of providers."[33]

Ron Schwartz, J.D., former deputy assistant inspector general of HHS, expressed his outrage that medical doctors are criminally prosecuted for overcharging by seven or nine dollars. Schwartz said that physicians who are overpaid should be penalized. However, he added:

> It's just an absolutely unbelievable thing to realize that all those cases, in which someone overcharged $7 or $9—all those cases are now criminal cases. That is an absolute disgrace to our country and a disgrace to our taxpayers to subsidize that.[34]

Schwartz emphasized that many physicians are guilty of "sloppy record keeping"; however, that does not justify charging them with criminal fraud.[35] He stressed that the government should not be in the business of "destroying professionals." Schwartz also explained that fraud investigators prefer criminal convictions over civil settlements because they get "more points" toward promotion by going for criminal convictions.[36] In addition, once the government gets a criminal conviction, it is relatively easy to also get a civil conviction and collect substantial fines from a physician. From the government's point of view, the criminal prosecution of doctors is a no-lose proposition.

Incredibly, Schwartz advises doctors who are wrongly accused of overbilling to "give them some money," or they will turn the case over to the IG for criminal prosecution. Ominously, he warns that federal investigators have "never walked away from a case because it was lousy."[37]

What Schwartz did not say, however, is that the extortion and malicious prosecution of medical doctors are a travesty of justice and a stain on the American system of justice. It is symptomatic of a larger problem: malevolent harassment or political persecution of a hallowed and honorable profession.

Edward J. Kuriansky, the deputy attorney general and chief of the Medicaid Fraud Control Unit of New York, was another enthusiastic champion of the IG's junkyard dog mentality. Kuriansky charged 200 doctors with criminal fraud of Medicaid. By 1990, Kuriansky achieved 155 convictions in 160 criminal cases. One case involved Dr. Eugeniu Liteanu, who was charged with five criminal felony counts of fraud involving $90 of alleged overbilling.

Dr. Liteanu was a 65-year-old Romanian-born psychiatrist with an unblemished 20-year record of professional service in New York. He had never been charged with malpractice, fraud, or abuse. The charges against him were based upon Dr. Liteanu's treatment of an undercover Medifraud investigator posing as a patient.

Eugeniu Liteanu billed Medicaid for complete therapy sessions when the investigator made excuses and cut short each session. There was nothing in the Medicaid guidelines on billing to cover psychiatric counseling sessions when a patient cuts them short. Nevertheless, Kuriansky justified the criminal indictment of Dr. Liteanu on his interpretation of Medicaid rules prohibiting a doctor from billing for sessions terminated by patients. He also offered the gratuitous remark that "Liteanu's profile" is consistent with that of a Medicaid cheat. He went on to elaborate:

> After considering the scope of Dr. Liteanu's alleged fraud (albeit small in dollar figures) as symptomatic of a far greater problem, the history and character of the defendant merely make him typical of the well-educated, often well-to-do, first-time offenders generally caught cheating the Medicaid program. Most taxpayers would support efforts to prosecute those who are accused of shortchanging the system.[38]

The Liteanu case illustrates the fact that antifraud investigators make up their own rules in order to indict physicians. The case also illustrates the fact that fraud investigators engage in profiling alleged perpetrators of health fraud: well-to-do, foreign-born physicians. Schwartz adds to this profile foreign medical graduates who practice in inner-city locations, are not board-certified, have a large number of Medicare or Medicaid patients, and are in solo practice.[39]

It is also clear that if there is any ambiguity surrounding a medical regulation or code, physicians will not be given the benefit of the doubt. Indeed, many innocent doctors have been fined millions and been sent to jail because of the government's arbitrary and vindictive interpretation of a vague code or regulation. Physicians cannot rely upon their constitutionally guaranteed right of presumption of innocence in a fraud case.

Donald Zerendow illustrated the lengths to which fraud investigators will go to get a criminal conviction of a physician. He recounted his experience defending a Massachusetts doctor with impeccable credentials and an unblemished 15-year record who was indicted for "massive fraud." Four months after the Massachusetts Medicaid Fraud Control Unit removed files from the doctor's office for a "routine audit," the physician was informed that he was going to be criminally indicted. They said that it had uncovered "massive" fraudulent billing for surgical procedures that other physicians in his specialty and locale did not perform.

Prosecutors claimed that the physician had overcharged the government by hundreds of thousands of dollars and that the doctor only had one alternative. That was to plead guilty to several felony counts and pay $150,000 in fines.

In exchange for the offer, the prosecutor said he would recommend a prison term of only three to five years.

Zerendow asked the prosecutors to show him the documentation for their charges against the physician. The prosecutor produced a thick computer printout that "showed" that the doctor's billings were "way off the charts."[40] They also said that this was the "best" fraud case that the prosecuting attorney had ever seen.

The prosecutors threatened that if the doctor did not accept their offer, they would convene a special grand jury and expand the criminal investigation to include the doctor's Medicare billings. They said that this would bring the IG's office into the case and would dramatically increase the doctor's financial penalties and jail time. According to Zerendow, the physician was essentially told:

> You can go to jail now or you can go to jail for a longer term later; pay us now or pay us more later. Look into your heart of hearts, doctor, and admit that you did wrong. Face up to your guilt and put this thing behind you.[41]

Zerendow told the doctor that this was a typical intimidation tactic that all fraud investigators used throughout the country. After much anguished thought, the physician decided to fight the charges.

As promised, the IG's office joined the criminal investigation. The investigative team traveled to every hospital and nursing home where the doctor treated patients. They interviewed well patients at their homes, elderly confined patients at bedside, hospital nurses, aides, orderlies, and administrators. The investigators took photographs and copied thousands of pages of records. They interviewed past and present employees. They searched the registry of deeds to determine the value of the doctor's real estate. They photographed the "for sale" sign at the physician's home, which he was forced to sell to meet lawyer's fees. Investigators interviewed the doctor's parents and asked a part-time employee at the physician's home if he was having marital problems.

In July 1988, the government's case against the physician was presented to the grand jury, and it indicted him on the following charges:

1. Between December 1983 and January 1987, the doctor received $369 from a Medicaid patient for services provided. However, Medicaid and not the patient should have been billed.
2. Between November 1984 and September 1987, the physician stole $2,600 from the Medicaid program.
3. Between December 1985 and December 1987, in 22 separate counts, the doctor stole a total of $430 from Medicaid.

After a two-year criminal investigation that cost the government over $100,000, it charged the physician with stealing $3,399 over a period of four years. Therefore, a case that was initially described as a "massive" fraud- ulent billing swindle became an allegation that the doctor had defrauded the government by $16.34 per week over four years.

On the day that the doctor was indicted, the prosecutor offered him a new deal. This offer was that the physician plead guilty to one felony count, pay the government $85,000 and serve six months in the penitentiary. The physician agonized again, but he decided to reject the offer and plead not guilty.

From this point on, the government's case unraveled. Three months after the indictment, the prosecutor dropped the first charge in the "interest of justice" because his sole witness was "delusional" and the government could not vouch for her credibility. The prosecution was also forced to drop the second charge because the disputed $2,600 was for services actually rendered by the physician but allegedly used the wrong CPT codes. The doctor petitioned the court for copies of the billing records and proved that he had, in fact, used the correct codes. The prosecutor never bothered even to check the CPT codes before criminally indicting the physician. On the final charge, overbilling Medicaid by $430, the prosecutor made still another offer. This offer was that the physician would reimburse Medicaid by $430, and pay $5,000 for the cost of the investigation, and agree not to participate in the Medicaid program. The doctor once again agonized over the offer but finally agreed to it after the prosecution added to the agreement that the physician had not violated any Medicaid regulation or any law.

Instead of being exonerated, however, and having his good name and property returned, the doctor was left bankrupt and without a home or assets. His professional reputation was destroyed by the criminal investigation.

Finally, in an act of vindictiveness, the IG excluded the doctor from the Medicare program on the specious grounds that the IG had the authority to exclude physicians who had been "suspended, excluded, or otherwise sanc- tioned." The IG's convoluted logic was that since the physician had withdrawn from Medicaid that constituted a "sanction" that justified the doctor's exclusion from Medicare for life.

Kusserow was also personally guilty of assassinating the characters of in- nocent physicians. In his eagerness to prosecute, fine, and exclude doctors from federally financed health programs, he vilified doctors. In one highly publicized episode, Kusserow made the statement that Dr. William Diefen- bach, M.D., a dedicated New York physician with an unblemished 20-year record of service, was excluded from Medicare on the grounds that he was a drug addict. Kusserow later retracted the statement; however, he insisted that Dr. Diefenbach should nevertheless be excluded from all federal programs because he was incompetent. The impact of Kusserow's public humiliation of Dr. Diefenbach was devastating. The doctor gave up his effort to restore his good name, sank deeply into depression, and committed suicide.

Despite the reign of terror that Kusserow unleashed upon many in- nocent physicians, he had powerful supporters in Congress. For example,

Representative Fortney "Pete" Stark (D-Calif.) described Kusserow in the following way:

> He is one of the toughest and best IGs in the federal government. Dick Kusserow should get a medal for saving the taxpayer fortunes. That he is being criticized today is a sure sign he is doing his job.[42]

Self-Perpetuating Fraud Bureaucracy

Richard Kusserow resigned as IG in June of 1992. He was placed under intensive pressure from 38 medical associations demanding that President George H. Bush remove him. The IG no longer uses numerical quotas as the basis for agents' promotion and pay increases. One might imagine, therefore, that the oppressive and criminally negligent behavior of the OIG under Krusserow had ended.

Unfortunately, however, this has not happened. In fact, just the opposite has occurred. In response to the explosive increase in the cost of government health programs, Congress passed the Health Insurance Portability and Accountability Act (HIPAA) of 1996. HIPAA has imposed heavier criminal and civil penalties for health fraud, made it easier to convict physicians of fraud, expanded criminal and civil laws to include private patients, and created a special fund for the purpose of financing additional health fraud investigations. The fund is called the Health Care Fraud and Abuse Control Program (HCFACP). Fines that are imposed upon physicians and other health providers are placed in this fund.

The fund is self-financing and unaccountable. In other words, the government's fraud investigation bureaucracy is financed by convictions of fraud. The more the number of convictions, the greater their budgetary resources. The purpose of the fund is to "create a powerful new criminal and civil enforcement tool to expand the fight against health care fraud."

The fund was placed under the control of the Attorney General and the secretary of the HHS. The Attorney General and secretary are empowered to allocate money recovered from health fraud fines and prosecutions to finance additional investigations and prosecutions of doctors. In other words, the government now has the resources and incentives to carry out unlimited investigations and prosecutions of physicians. Indeed, funding for the fraud bureaucracy depends upon income derived from new investigations and prosecutions. This self-perpetuating bureaucracy depends upon the prosecution of more and more doctors and providers whether justified or not. Indeed, if their mission was achieved and health fraud declined, the reason for the existence of a health fraud bureaucracy would disappear.

Table 3.1 shows the amount of money the federal government has recovered from HCFACP-financed investigations from 1998 to 2002. It increased

Table 3.1
Money Recovered by HCFACP-Financed OIG Investigations (Dollars in
Thousands)

	1998	2000	2002	2005
Gift-bequests	$3	$6	$7	$30,863
Criminal fines	$2,503	$57,209	$430,536	$347,896
Civil fines	$1,855	$147,268	$6,693	$13,435
False Claims Act	$103,026	$37,400	$328,566	$347,896
Audit recover	$144,742	NA	$150,571	$423,335
Defense Department	$7,489	$2,514	$12,537	$3,351
Personnel management	$174	$7,570	$50,571	$4,003
OIG of HHS	$1,270	$2,890	NA	$9,433
Other agencies	$3,125	$9,350	NA	$1,314
Relators' payments (whistleblowers)	$4,345	$90,027	$101,165	$136,757
Total[a]	$296,531	$717,156	$1,631,621	$1,708,959

Note: [a]Includes miscellaneous spending for administration and related expenses. Funds were also collected on behalf of state Medicaid programs and private insurance companies. These funds are not included in the totals. The government acknowledges that over $3 billion annually is actually recovered.
Source: Annual Reports of HHS and the Department of Justice on the Health Care Fraud and Abuse Control Program, 1998–2006.

from $296 million in 1998 to more than $1.7 billion in 2005. That figure does not include Medicaid or private insurance money collected by the government, however. When that money is added, the figure rises to over $3 billion dollars a year.

Table 3.2 shows how HCFACP funds were allocated for additional investigations and prosecutions. HCFACP funding increased from $175 million in 1998 to more than $240 million in 2005. The number of fraud investigators in the OIG of HHS increased by 40 percent from 1998 to 2005. In 1998, there were 260 auditors and 136 criminal investigators. In 2006, there were 1500 investigators and attorneys.

HCFACP provides funding for the 93 USAOs throughout the country and FBI field agents for health fraud enforcement. FBI health fraud investigations increased by more than 400 percent from 591 in 1992 to 2,547 cases in 2005. FBI agents also coordinate health care fraud task forces including state and local law enforcement agencies and private insurance fraud investigators.

For every dollar spent on health fraud investigation and prosecution, the government gets more than five dollars back in fines and penalties. In 2001, more than 2,000 defendants were convicted for health fraud offenses, and over 15,000 were excluded from Medicare, Medicaid, and other health care

Table 3.2
HCFACP Funds Allocated for Health Fraud Investigations (Dollars in Thousands)

	1998	2000	2002	2005
OIG of HHS	$85,680	$119,250	$145,000	$160,000
OIG General Counsel	$2,200	$1,949	$4,180	$4,778
Administration on Aging	$1,300	$1,450	$2,000	$3,128
Health Resources Services Admin.	$1,000	$396	$2,675	$450
HCFA/CMS	$950	$55	$125	$22,297
U.S. Attorneys	$23,856	$23,150	$25,200	$30,400
Civil Division	$3,803	$10,751	$26,029	$14,459
Criminal Division	$561	$827	$1,270	$1,580
Justice Management Division	$250	$343	$886[a]	NA
FBI	$56,000	$76,000	$101,000	$114,000
Total[a]	*$175,600*	*$234,171*	*$310,180*	*$240,558*

Note: [a]Includes miscellaneous administrative expenses.
Source: Annual Reports of HHS and the Department of Justice on the Health Care Fraud and Abuse Control Program, 1998–2006.

programs. From October 2004 to June 2006, the IG has won 760 criminal convictions, 381 civil actions, and more than 5,300 doctors and other medical professionals were prohibited from treating Medicare and Medicaid patients—3,448 were excluded for crimes against Medicare and Medicaid and the licenses of more than 1,720 doctors were revoked.

An Antifraud Industry

In order to maintain their jobs and receive promotions and pay raises, therefore, auditors, investigators, and prosecutors must find new cases of medical fraud. The fraud bureaucracy's need for increasing sources of funding is confirmed in an interview with Wayne W. Oakes, the acting chief of the FBI's health care fraud unit. In response to the question, "Will you ever reach a point where you have enough agents?" Oakes made the following remark:

> I don't think so because what happens here is when you fund, say 46 positions, and you use part or most of that, what happens is the cost of that agent increases each year because there are promotions involved.[43]

Oakes pointed out that investigations are increasingly more sophisticated. He noted that it is expensive, for example, to carry out 35 search warrants in 17 states with box loads of records that have to be stored. The insurance companies work closely with snitches and whistleblowers to document fraud allegations against physicians. The companies have their own internal fraud control units that audit physicians' billing records and provide the evidence needed by law enforcement agencies to fine and prosecute doctors. Once insurers establish what they believe is evidence of fraud, they refer the case to the USAO or other law enforcement agencies.

The federal government is only too happy to audit cases of alleged fraud. They have a so-called "formula" for financial returns on their audits. They expected to receive a monetary return of five to one or six to one on their audits.

In other words, if an insurance company spends $5,000 auditing a physician's Medicare or Medicaid billing, the government expects to receive between $25,000 and $30,000 in recovered fines from the doctor. For this reason, much of the evidence used by prosecutors to fine, indict, and try physicians is produced by insurance companies.

As is the case with whistleblowers, the insurance companies are also rewarded financially by receiving a portion of the fines levied against doctors. Likewise, under the terms of the Comprehensive Forfeiture Act of 1984, law enforcement agencies can seize a physician's assets, including property, and retain a portion of it for their own use. This occurs without any hearing or trial. All that is needed is "probable cause" or suspicion that a crime was committed.

The upshot of this for many innocent physicians is that they are denied the use of their own assets to pay for defense counsel and must rely upon the second-rate quality of public defenders. Many doctors receive the same quality of justice meted out to indigents accused of violent street crimes. Indeed, they may not even receive a defense of that quality because few criminal defense attorneys have the expertise, time, or interest to master the complexities of medical law.

In effect, the government has created a powerful economic incentive for all those close to medical doctors to have them investigated and charged with fraud. This lays the groundwork for extortion and medical McCarthyism by snitches, whistleblowers, insurance companies, the federal government, and law enforcement agencies. The elimination of health fraud would mean the elimination of jobs, financial rewards, and seized property. This has created a vicious cycle of prosecutions with potentially devastating consequences for many innocent doctors.

4

PROSECUTING DOCTORS: SEXUAL HARASSMENT PAYBACK AND CREATING CRIMES

The Department of Justice (DOJ) embarked upon a major new law enforcement policy in 1993. It shifted its priorities from multinational drug cartels and the Savings and Loan scandals to health care fraud. The department created a Health Care Fraud Subcommittee under the Attorney General's Advisory Committee to carry out the new policy. The subcommittee was comprised of representatives from each of the 93 United States Attorney Generals' Offices (USAOs) throughout the country. The job of the subcommittee was to coordinate the government's war on health fraud, the new number-one white-collar crime.

The first step in this war was to identify, depersonalize, and give a negative image to the enemy: "The healthcare fraud industry."[1] This term was first used in 1995 in the *USA Bulletin*, which is the Justice Department's professional journal. The DOJ's objective was to stigmatize medical professionals with the same public hostility that is associated with corporate crimes such as "insider-trading" on Wall Street and owners of failed S&Ls. Prosecutors throughout the country sent in war stories and lessons learned in indicting and prosecuting physicians and other providers.

Prosecutors were given vast resources and powers to prosecute health care criminals. As in the case of a real war, prosecutors must have enough power to do their jobs, however, not so much power that they threaten the careers and lives of innocent doctors.

James V. Smith correlates the arrogant and cocky attitude of some health care prosecutors with the Tom Cruise character in the movie "Top Gun."[2] In the film, Cruise was a member of an elite team of highly skilled and daring pilots. However, his risky behavior was dangerous to other pilots and to their mission.

Prosecutors who are given too much power may also become arrogant and dangerous. In their eagerness to get convictions, they may cast their nets too widely and prosecute blameless physicians. When doctors' careers are destroyed by unfair accusations, prosecutions become persecutions.

"RIGHT STUFF" FOR HEALTH CARE PROSECUTORS

In a *USA Bulletin* published in April 1997, two assistant United States' Attorneys and a DOJ trial attorney discuss the "right stuff" for health care prosecutors.[3] The title of the article is "The Tao of the Health Care Fraud Trial." The prosecutors explain their health fraud trial strategy by making reference to the ancient Chinese religion of Taoism and Sun Tzu's 2,500-year-old classic book on warfare called *The Art of Warfare.*

From Taoism, they took the principle of a single unity behind the bewildering multiplicity and contradictions of life to explain health fraud to a jury. From Sun Tzu, they took the military strategy that "victory comes not to the stronger or more courageous, but to he who chooses his ground well, and draws his opponent into joining the battle."[4]

This military analogy not only reveals a contempt for a just verdict in health fraud trials, but it exposes an arrogant and cocky attitude comparable to the Cruise character in "Top Gun." Several passages from the article will illustrate this.

They refer to health care fraud prosecutions as the "Golden Goose."[5] They say that health fraud cases differ from most criminal cases in that there is a question that a crime actually occurred. An impartial observer would have to wonder why such cases would ever go to trial in the first place.

Instead of undertaking the difficult task of proving that physicians violated Byzantine and ambiguous billing regulations, prosecutors take the easier path of placing the tainted public image of doctors on trial. In fact, the authors attribute their success

> to competent and spectacularly energetic criminal investigators' instinct for recognizing the larcenous spirit in perpetrators.[6]

In other words, prosecutors rely upon criminal investigators to produce evidence of a defendant's dishonest nature. Anything investigators can find to suggest that a physician performed medical services for financial gain reinforces jurors' predisposition to convict doctors of fraud. This includes an affluent lifestyle. The following statement illustrates this line of reasoning.

> (A doctor) enjoys a lifestyle which the average juror will find difficult to reconcile with honest business practices.

The implication is that it is unethical or unseemly for physicians to be prosperous. Prosecutors elaborate this theme of callous and uncaring doctors.

> Most jurors have waited many frustratingly long mornings to see a doctor, have been shabbily and impersonally handled by clinics and emergency rooms, and have fought nearly to tears to get insurance or benefit payments for essential

medical care, guaranteeing them a predisposition to take full advantage of their jury service to return the favor to the authors of their ire, who are conveniently seated at the defense table.[7]

They emphasize the importance of "defining the defendant as an aggrandizing schemer engaged in self-enriching fraud."[8] According to the prosecutors, "blessedly" there are "badges of fraud" such as omission of information and false or misleading statements in patients' charts or billing records that can be used to convict doctors.

If the prosecution bases its case upon a technical violation of billing regulations, they add badges of fraud to the charges to simplify the case for the jury. When the prosecution's evidence does not fit any criminal statue, they use "mental nimbleness" to detect what they call a "pattern of (*fraudulent*) activity." Prosecutors routinely use "elastic" criminal statutes such as mail and wire fraud and money laundering to fit the "pattern of activity."[9]

This explains the fact that hundreds of charges are typically brought against physicians in fraud cases. Even if doctors are declared innocent of most of the charges, the sheer number of accusations encourages jurors to believe that physicians are guilty of something. Hence, most doctors who are tried for fraud are found guilty of at least a few felony charges.

Energetic criminal investigation, mental nimbleness, persistence, and an instinct for recognizing the "larcenous spirit" in human nature may be the "right stuff" for successful health fraud prosecutors. However, it often results in destroying the careers and lives of innocent doctors.

Sexual Harassment Payback: Dr. Patsy M. Vargo

In 1996, Patsy Vargo became a victim of the government's war on medical doctors after a 15-year career as a dedicated rural family doctor in Montana. Dr. Vargo was an attractive and popular 38-year-old petite physician. She was the daughter of a Presbyterian minister of Scottish background with the maiden name Mackintosh. Vargo lived with her husband, Frank, and their three teenage children in a refurbished two-bedroom ranch home rebuilt by her husband. The ranch nested in rolling hills between Selby and Conrad. It was 80 miles from the nearest city, Great Falls. Patsy Vargo had a small solo practice in Great Falls, while her husband worked on the ranch.

In 1989, Dr. Vargo was offered a position at the Malmstrom Air Force Base's 341st Strategic Clinic in Great Falls, Montana, primarily to treat female dependents of retired military personnel. The patients were in the Civilian Health and Medical Program of the Uniformed Services (CHAMPUS). Military doctors could not handle the growing number of retired military dependents in the area.

They asked Dr. Vargo to join the clinic because she was a woman and had a special interest in gynecological and geriatric care. She started working at the clinic two or three days a week but soon became so popular with patients that she closed her private practice in Great Falls and started working full time at the base.

From 1989 till 1996, Patsy Vargo was the most sought after physician at the clinic, averaging 30 to 40 patients a day compared to about 12 patients a day for Air Force doctors. Vargo was so prolific that she became one of the busiest CHAMPUS doctors in the country. Patsy Vargo uniformly received excellent ratings by her military supervisors, and her billing practices were used by clinic administrators as the standard to evaluate other civilian doctors at the clinic.

Indeed, during this period, the contracts of several civilian doctors were not renewed because they billed for services that were not performed. For example, an audit of Dr. John Belt's billing records in 1993 turned up irregularities; however, he was allowed to resign in 1995. No charges were ever brought against him.

Patsy Vargo's circumstances altered dramatically after a change in command at the clinic. In 1993, Major Timothy K. Guthrie replaced Major John Highsmith as the Chief of Professional Services in the clinic. The Chief of Professional Services is responsible for oversight of the civilian doctors at the clinic. This includes reviewing patient charts. Just before Highsmith was reassigned, he made the following statement about Patsy Vargo's performance at the clinic.

> Dr. Vargo's patient care was uniformly excellent. Vargo was a harder worker than most, stayed late to see patients was quite efficient despite the inbred inefficiencies of the practice of military medicine. There was never any indication that she "cheated" in any way, billed for patients she didn't actually care for. If the issue is that she didn't comply with requirements of the government, that issue is bogus.[10]

Initially, Guthrie and the other military doctors were pleased with the quality of Dr. Vargo's medical care. Indeed, many of them, including Guthrie, chose her to be their family physician.

In late 1994, however, all of that changed. Two military doctors at the clinic were charged with sexual harassment. Dr. Timothy Guthrie and Dr. Jon Walz were accused of sexual harassment because of racial-sexual comments they made to a beautiful black secretary named Monica R. Lancot who was a civil service employee at the clinic. Colonel Ken Rashid, the commander of the clinic, was also criticized for not stopping the harassment. The secretary was one of Dr. Vargo's patients and confided in her that she was under extreme stress due to her employers' behavior. Lancot explained that Guthrie and Walz repeatedly made offensive sexual-racial jokes in Lancot's presence and asked that she include them in the minutes of morning staff meetings. She was instructed to repeat the jokes to them by reading the minutes out loud while they laughed. She was then ordered to delete the jokes.

Lancot went to Dr. Vargo and requested prescriptions for Prozac or valium or anything that would make her work more tolerable. She did not want to lose her seniority in the civil service but at the same time felt humiliated. Lancot filed harassment charges against the officers, and an Air Force hearing was convened in January of 1995 to consider the charges.

Since the secretary had confided in Dr. Vargo, the judge advocate's staff asked her to testify at the harassment hearing. Vargo feared the repercussions of testifying against Air Force doctors, but was told by the judge advocate's staff that if she refused to meet with them, her contract with the Air Force would be cancelled. Vargo reluctantly gave a deposition in January 1995. Her taped testimony occurred in the legal office on base at 7:00 A.M. and was subsequently used at the harassment hearing.

Following the hearing, the doctors were given a verbal reprimand. All three were transferred from Malmstrom ABF in mid-1995. Colonel Rashid was reassigned to New Mexico and later left the Air Force, Dr. Walz left active duty service but stayed in the Air Force reserves, and Major Guthrie was sent to Germany. However, instead of damaging Guthrie's career, he was promoted to lieutenant colonel in May 1995 and to full colonel in 2001.

Retaliation for Testifying

On the evening of February 19, 1995, Dr. Jon Walz, an Air Force physician at the clinic and a friend of Major Guthrie, called Vargo at her home. Walz said that he had just come from the Air Force Office of Special Investigations (AFOSI) at Malmstrom Air Force Base and told Vargo that her billing records were being investigated and she would "lose her license, go to jail, and never practice medicine again."[11]

On March 16, 1995, the Office of Special Investigations (AFOSI) at Malmstrom Air Force Base, led by agent Carlos Vargas, transmitted Guthrie and Walz's accusations of Dr. Vargo to Special Agent Gary A. Pacey of the Defense Department's Criminal Investigative Service (DCIS) of the Inspector General office based in Seattle.[12] DCIS and the U.S. Air Force Office of Special Investigations at Malmstrom Air Force Base conducted a joint investigation of Dr. Vargo.

On April 4, 1995, agents Vargas and Pacey visited the 341st Medical Support Squadron at Malmstrom Air Force Base where they met with Major Guthrie, Dr. Walz, Lieutenant Colonel Thomas Leach, Colonel Rashid and others. Guthrie turned over Dr. Vargo's internal audit records to the investigators. The audit of Dr. Vargo was originally ordered by Major Guthrie and carried out by Lieutenant Colonel Thomas Leach, M.D. Guthrie chose Leach for this task because he had a civilian practice before joining the Air Force, and, therefore, had some knowledge of CPT billing codes. Leach also had free time to do the audit because he had been suspended from treating patients because of complaints. According to Dr. Vargo, Leach was told that if he did a good job on the audit, he would be given an honorable discharge from the Air Force.

Leach obtained billing records from CHAMPUS for Dr. Vargo and four other civilian doctors for the period of February 1993 to August 1994. This was the first time such an audit had been done at the clinic. Dr. Leach compared Vargo's billing profile with the four other civilian doctors at the clinic. He found that Dr. Vargo billed CHAMPUS at higher CPT codes than the other doctors. For example, the report stated:

> Dr. Vargo billed approximately 52 percent of her claims at the 99214 CPT code rate, over 18 percent at the 99215 CPT code rate and less than 8 percent at the 99213 CPT code for the 1993–1994. Another civilian doctor billed about 50 percent of his claims at the 99213 CPT code rate, 19 percent at the 99214 CPT code rate and less than 1 percent at the 99215 CPT code rate.[13]

Leach's audit of Dr. Vargo merely confirmed what everyone already knew. Patsy Vargo was not only the busiest doctor at the clinic but she took the most difficult cases involving the greatest complexity and therefore requiring the highest billing codes. Nevertheless, Major Guthrie and Dr. Walz gave the audit of Dr. Vargo to investigators as evidence of her criminal behavior.

Government Investigation and Indictment

In late February 1995, Dr. Vargo confronted both Guthrie and Walz about the warning she had been given. They responded that they were duty bound to report any fraudulent billing to authorities. They said that they had reported her up-coding to the Office of Special Investigations at Malstrom AFB. They also sent a copy of the complaint to the Defense Criminal Investigation Services of the Inspector General's Office in the Department of Defense.

Dr. Vargo asked the clinic commander, Dr. Ken Rashid, if there were any problems with her billing, and he reassured her that there were none and she should keep up her excellent work at the clinic.[14] Indeed, complaints of Dr. Vargo's alleged up-coding completely circumvented Air Force regulations for handling billing irregularities. Aberrations must be reported first to the Executive Committee of the clinic, chaired at the time by Dr. Rashid. The investigation of Dr. Vargo was never reported to the Executive Committee of the clinic despite the fact that fraud investigators interviewed all members of the committee. Major Guthrie and Dr. Walz went outside the normal Air Force procedures in reporting Dr. Vargo for fraudulent billing.

They not only circumvented the chain of command, but Patsy Vargo was the only civilian physician at Malmstrom AFB who has ever been turned in for fraudulent billing. This was despite the fact that several other doctors were audited and found to be billing for services not rendered. They were allowed to resign without penalties or investigation. One must ask, why Patsy Vargo? This is especially troublesome given the fact that she was the most efficient and popular physician at the clinic.

The Investigation

The lead investigator in Dr. Vargo's case was Special Agent Gary A. Pacey of the DCIS. Pacey was based in Seattle and worked on the case with Special Agent Carlos Vargas, who was based at Malmstrom AFB.

At 9:00 P.M. on February 28, 1996, Pacey and Vargas went to Dr. Vargo's home wearing gun holsters, badges, and trench coats to serve a subpoena ordering her to appear before a federal grand jury. The subpoena demanded that she turn over 62,000 copies of her billing records covering eight years of her practice at Malmstrom AFB to Assistant U.S. Attorney, Carl E. Rostad. It cost Vargo more than $5,000 to copy the documents, which were delivered in a truck. Outraged by this action, Patsy Vargo immediately resigned from Malmstrom AFB.

When agent Pacey was later asked by Vargo's attorney why all the cloak and dagger activity? Why scare the family and children? Why not confront the accused alone at work? He said that "we wanted the element of surprise, we wanted to intimidate her."[15]

Rogstad worked closely with Pacey in putting together a criminal case against Vargo. After combing through Vargo's billing records for two and a half years, they succeeded in getting her indicted by a federal grand jury. On June 19, 1997, Patsy Vargo was indicted on two felony counts. One was defrauding the federal government by "up-coding" her billing statement to the government, and the other was mail fraud. She was indicted for mail fraud because the bills she submitted to Medicare through Palmetto Government Benefits Administrators, an affiliate of Blue Cross and Blue Shield, were sent via U.S. mail. If convicted, Dr. Vargo could have been given a prison sentence of 10 years and/or a $500,000 fine.

In the process of the investigation, Dr. Vargo was denied due process of the law. She was indicted without being interviewed by federal investigators. They also did not interview material witnesses to her innocence. This included Major Larry Thornhill, who was the clinic administrator and finance director from July 1990 to July 1993.

On numerous occasions, Dr. Vargo sought to meet with Rogstad to explain any billing irregularities. Rogstad refused, however, insisting that she meet with the investigators, Pacey and Vargas. Furthermore, Rogstad took the position that the investigators would meet with her only to discuss the "pattern of (*fraudulent*) billing" without getting into particular cases.[16] Dr. Vargo, on the other hand, wanted to discuss specific cases of alleged fraudulent billing. She argued that it was unreasonable to expect her to be conversant with thousands of cases several years old without the opportunity to review them in advance.

Prosecutors refused her request, however, arguing that the element of surprise and spontaneity was an important part of criminal interviews. They finally agreed to meet with Vargo after the indictment, however. The meeting occurred on June 27, 1997. Patsy Vargo was astonished to hear Carl Rogstad accuse her face to face of lying. He said: "You are just like every other criminal. You're incredibly convincing and a huge liar. I don't believe a word you said."[17]

The indictment was based upon an egregious misinterpretation of CPT codes. Prosecutors claimed that the reimbursement for a physician was based solely upon the time spent with patients. The indictment was, therefore, based upon the time required for "face-to-face" contact with patients. They supplied the following office CPT codes, the level of complexity, and the time associated with each to prove their point.

Office Visits	Minutes
Established Patient	
CPT Code 99211 (minimal problem)	5
CPT Code 99212 (minor problem)	10
CPT Code 99213 (moderate problem)	15
CPT Code 99214 (moderate-severe)	25
CPT Code 99215 (moderate-high severe)	40
New Patient	
CPT Code 99201 (minor problem)	10
CPT Code 99202 (moderate-low severe)	20
CPT Code 99203 (moderate problem)	30
CPT Code 99204 (moderate-high severe)	45
CPT Code 99205 (moderate-high severe)	60

For example, 59 percent of Dr. Vargo's claims were coded as 99214 (established patient with moderate-severe problems), requiring 25 minutes of face-to-face time. In fact, she spent on average only 10 minutes with these patients. According to the government's interpretation of the codes, Vargo should have coded these claims as 99212 (minor problems). They also claimed that CPT codes 99211 and 99201 required 5 and 10 minutes, respectively, of a physician's face-to-face contact with a patient. In fact, these codes do not require any direct patient contact with a doctor.

The U.S. Attorney claimed that Dr. Vargo devised a fraudulent scheme to obtain money by deliberately using CPT codes that required more time than she actually spent treating patients. The government added up all the minutes for the CPT codes that Dr. Vargo billed the government and concluded that it would amount to 15 to 24 hours of "face-to-face" time per day. Since that was physically impossible, Rogstad concluded that Dr. Vargo had cheated the government by "up-coding" her claims.

Malicious Interpretation of Codes

The government completely ignored its own expert witness in the case, Glenn D. Littenberg, M.D., PAC, and proceeded with its indictment of Dr. Vargo based upon a bogus interpretation of CPT codes. The U.S. Attorney hired Littenberg as its expert witness to evaluate Dr. Vargo's alleged "up-coding." Littenberg was a doctor of internal medicine and gastroenterology in

Pasadena, California, and a nationally renowned expert on coding regulations. He also served on the AMA's committee on CPT coding.

After examining Dr. Vargo's patient charts and billing records, Littenberg said that the government's criminal case against Vargo was groundless and "did not hold any weight at all."[18] This conclusion was reinforced by a letter from the American Academy of Family Physicians. The letter explained that CPT codes for office visits (called Evaluation and Management, or E/M) should be selected on the basis of seven components: history, examination, medical decision-making, counseling, coordination of care, nature of presenting problem, and lastly, time.[19]

The first three components—history, examination, and medical decision-making—are the key elements in deciding the appropriate CPT billing code. Time is a factor in cases only where counseling or coordination of care involves more than 50 percent of the physician-patient encounter. Since most of Dr. Vargo's cases involved difficult gynecological diseases and geriatric treatment, time was not an important factor in her CPT codes.

Office codes have "typical times" associated with them; however, they are average times. There is a wide range of time physicians spend with patients depending upon their efficiency and productivity. A highly efficient and busy doctor such as Patsy Vargo requires less time in performing gynecological exams, for example, than a physician who seldom performs such examinations. Indeed, many family physicians do not even provide this kind of care.

Everyone agreed that Pasty Vargo was an extraordinarily efficient and productive physician capable of treating large numbers of patients. Dr. Vargo scheduled patients from 8:00 A.M. to 6:00 P.M. every day and worked through her lunch hour. Air Force physicians devoted a full hour for all minor procedures, whereas Dr. Vargo saw a patient every 15 to 30 minutes. She was booked up months in advance but always made room for urgent walk-in patients. In fact, the janitorial staff was upset that they could not clean up the clinic because Dr. Vargo stayed very late to see patients.

Air Force doctors frequently attended meetings and training programs that would last an entire day. Patsy Vargo not only saw more patients than any other doctor at the clinic, but also she took the difficult patients who were time-consuming because of their complicated and conflicting diseases. When Patsy Vargo resigned from the clinic in 1996 and started a private practice in Shelby, Montana, most of her patients went with her. They preferred to travel 70 miles from Great Falls to be treated by Dr. Vargo than return to the clinic.

Major Terry Ryan, M.D., an Air Force physician at the clinic who worked with Dr. Vargo for five years before he retired made the following statement.

When we discovered the Air Force was unjustly persecuting an outstanding physician like Dr. Vargo, we knew that our decision (*to retire*) was for the best. I am enclosing this plaque (*of commendation*) with my letter. I now only see it as a symbol of injustice.[20]

Change of Prosecutorial Strategy

The government dropped its criminal indictment of Dr. Vargo on December 1, 1997. However, the U.S. Attorney, Sherry Scheel Matteucci, said that she would refer the case to the civil enforcement division of the USAO for possible prosecution. This was a canard, however. In effect, she took the case from one of her office assistants, Carl Rogstad, and handed to another assistant, Leif M. Johnson, for prosecution. The case never left her office or her authority.

Matteucci's objective was unchanged; it was just an adjustment in strategy. They felt that they could more easily convict Dr. Vargo under civil charges than criminal charges. Apparently, no serious thought was given to whether she was actually guilty of anything.

Indeed, Matteucci's appointment to the Attorney General's elite advisory council made it almost inevitable that she would make a second attempt to convict Patsy Vargo. Furthermore, her other assistant, Leif M. Johnson, had recently won a huge civil case against a Great Falls clinic charging that it had billed for more patients than it is physically possible in a day. They were encouraged to believe, therefore, that they could convict Dr. Vargo.

In January 1999, the government threatened Dr. Vargo with prosecution under the feared False Claims Act. The False Claims Act is a particularly odious law that prosecutors use to terrify innocent doctors. The law was originally enacted in 1863 to combat rampant fraud committed by the Union Army during the civil war.

In 1986, it was amended to eliminate the requirement to prove intent to defraud. This effectively shifted the burden of proof from the government to the defendant. The defendant was now guilty until proven innocent. The fines were also increased from two to three times the total damages, plus the fine for each individual fraudulent claim was increased from $2,000 to $10,000.

The threat of invoking the False Claims Act was designed to coerce Dr. Vargo into pleading guilty to fraud and paying a huge fine. In 1999, the government offered to settle the case if Patsy Vargo would plead guilty to false claims and pay a fine of $300,000. Johnson said that a conservative estimate of the government's overpayments to Dr. Vargo was between $125,000 and $175,000. The U.S. Attorney wanted to collect that amount plus the cost of the investigation.[21]

Patsy Vargo was dismayed and angered, however. She continued to deny any wrongdoing and was infuriated that the government would demand money from her to settle a case of wrongful prosecution. After all, she was the injured party, with legal expenses of more than $500,000.

Prosecution under the False Claims Act

On December 2, 1999, exactly two years after the government dropped its criminal indictment, it again filed charges against Patsy Vargo, this time under the False Claims Act. The evidence for the charges was audits conducted by two physicians at the Malstrom AFB clinic in 1995 and 1996.

The government used an October 1994 audit performed by Dr. Thomas Leach's audit to charge Dr. Vargo. Leach's audit is flawed insofar as he took a statistically unrepresentative 10 percent sample of Patsy Vargo's claims and reported that Vargo had up-coded every one of the 280 claims she submitted from November 14, 1994 to December 13, 1994.

On May 8, 1996, agents Pacey and Vargas met with Colonel Dr. Lopez, the chief of Medical Services at Malmstrom AFB and Major Guthrie's replacement, to discuss what "we needed the doctors to do" in the investigation of Dr. Vargo.[22] Colonel Lopez asked Dr. Howard P. Blount, another civilian physician at the clinic, to evaluate 175 of Dr. Vargo's claims. The sample of claims was also statistically unrepresentative. Based on these claims, Blount reported that 56 of the 175 claims were up-coded, 9 lacked adequate documentation or billed for a new patient CPT code instead of an established one. Extrapolating from this data, the government estimated that from 1991 to 1995, Dr. Vargo had fraudulently billed for 7,400 CPT codes. The penalty for up-coding was at least $5,000 for each false claim, amounting to a colossal fine of $37 million.

The evidence for Vargo's up-coding, however, was just as weak as it was in the criminal indictment. Neither Leach or Blount had any expertise in CPT coding. When Blount was asked about his qualifications to audit Dr. Vargo's billing records, for example, he said, that "I went in the military so I would not have to deal with them."[23] Indeed, Dr. Blount had minimal training in CPT coding. He attended only two brief training seminars given by military personnel in Alaska and at Malmstrom. Even more serious was the state of recordkeeping at the base. Richard A. Gordon, an investigator at Malmstrom, said that "nearly half of the billing records are not available." He observed that he was "skeptical and nervous" about the incomplete records and made the following comment:

> These records could conceivably cloudy the water if the defendant found out about it. She has many friends at the hospital that could tell her about this.[24]

John W. Osment, the Chief Information Officer at Malmstrom AFB acknowledged the problem by using the old adage, "garbage in, garbage out" and said that "the use of this bogus information was neither uncommon or isolated to Dr. Vargo."[25]

Indeed, the government's own coding expert, Dr. Littenberg, was so outraged by the continued prosecution of Dr. Vargo that he joined Patsy Vargo's defense team.

Littenberg made the following statement:

> I was greatly surprised and dismayed to hear that the criminal charges against Dr. Vargo were dropped subsequent to my 1997 report, only to be pursued under the False Claims Act, particularly after my opinion then, as it remains now, that there is no basis for the government's claims.[26]

Littenberg criticized the government's unscientific comparison of Dr. Vargo's billing charts with a tiny handful of unknown physicians in Colorado. The government did not follow statistically appropriate sampling techniques, did not reveal the nature of the other doctors' patient base, nor provided their patient charts for evaluation.

The government also used two nonphysician coding experts who concluded that Dr. Vargo did not provide adequate documentation in patients' charts to justify high-level CPT codes. However, these auditors used CPT documentation requirements that were not in use at the time that Patsy Vargo coded patient visits.

Littenberg compared Patsy Vargo's predicament to a motorist who, two and a half years after crossing an intersection, is told that a stop sign exists at an intersection and the motorist is guilty of running the sign.

Victory without Vindication

At a federal pretrial hearing in federal court on April 19, 2000, the government was forced to admit that it did not even have the military medical charts necessary to substantiate Dr. Vargo's fraud. Assistant U.S. Attorney Lief Johnson revealed that Vargo's records were spread all over the world. Nevertheless, he asked the judge for more time to investigate Dr. Vargo further. The judge reluctantly granted the request; however, he warned him to "quit fishing and cut bait."

After the government made several more attempts to prove that Dr. Vargo was guilty of fraud, it finally gave up its six-year-long prosecution of Patsy Vargo. On July 23, 2001, the U.S. District Court for Montana dismissed all charges against Dr. Vargo. However, at that hearing, Patsy Vargo insisted upon her innocence and said that she wanted complete exoneration. The judge threatened her by saying that if she insisted upon pursuing the case, it could drag on for years and add to her already crippling legal costs.

Indeed, he said that even if she won the case, any restitution she might receive would pale compared to the costs of her continued legal defense. Furthermore, the judge ordered Dr. Vargo to sign a gag order to prevent her from even discussing the terms of the settlement. Patsy Vargo was already financially devastated and reluctantly agreed to the settlement to put the issue behind her and get on with her and her children's lives.

This was a hollow victory for Patsy Vargo. Her six-year nightmare was over, but it cost her dearly. She was saddled with a huge legal bill of more than $350,000; she lost the ranch she loved; she suffered a debilitating illness that reduced her lung capacity by half; she lost her marriage of 20 years; and her teenage children were forced to grow up in the shadow of fear and disgrace of government investigation and harassment.

INSURANCE COMPANIES CREATE CRIMES: DR. ALLAN D. BELDEN

Dr. Allan "Luke" Belden was a 62-year-old physician and psychiatrist in solo practice in Appleton, Wisconsin, when the government targeted him for prosecution in 1999. Luke Belden was raised, along with two sisters, in Minot, North Dakota. His father was a traveling sales representative selling meat to grocery store butchers covering large areas of North Dakota and making $2,600 a year. Luke Belden saw his father only on weekends. The family later moved to Red Wing, Minnesota; where his father came home at night after work. Luke would accompany his father at 9:30 P.M. to the train station to mail the daily meat orders.

The family was poor, and Belden slept on a couch downstairs in the living room of their small farm home. He did not have his own furniture and shared one drawer of his sister's chest upstairs in the bathroom. He began working at age 13 and never asked for nor received financial support from his parents. In high school he had one pair of jeans and a flannel shirt, which he washed and ironed every day in preparation for school.

At age 15, he got a job cleaning and doing minor repairs at a 15-cabin lodge operation. With the money he put aside, plus earnings from a variety of janitorial and construction jobs, Luke managed to save enough during the summers and school breaks to buy his parents an electric refrigerator, phono-graph, and a small, used, black-and-white TV. Luke Belden could easily have been a hero in one of Horatio Alger's books. He was the embodiment of Alger's idols: he was religious, moral, brave, generous, kind, diligent, industri-ous, and persevering.

As a senior in high school, Belden was the manager of the school band, made the National Honor Society, played defensive end in football, had the lead in the senior class play, and took second place in the Minnesota state 880-yard run. He graduated from high school in 1954 and entered premedical studies at the University of Minnesota. In his second year of college, he was selected as one of six students in the country to study premedicine abroad at the American University of Beirut by the Board of Foreign Missions of the Presbyterian Church. After a year, he returned to America on a boat filled with World Council of Churches "work-campers" where he met his future wife Mary, who was a sophomore at Wellesley College.

Luke returned to the University of Minnesota and they corresponded by mail. In 1959, during his second year in medical school, they married after being together physically for only 13 days. Belden later explained his rush to marry. It was a rebound to a traumatic experience he had in medical school when his pathology professor drugged and sodomized him after a party in his home. Luke felt debased and humiliated and felt he had to prove that he was not homosexual.

Luke graduated fifth in his medical school class in 1961. This was despite his lifelong difficulty concentrating; his condition was later diagnosed as Attention Deficit Hyperactivity Disorder (ADHD). ADHD is a neurological disorder that affects between 3 and 5 percent of the U.S. population. It causes distractibility, forgetfulness, and disorganization. For example, when Luke studied at the medical library, he used a timer, setting it for 20 minutes.

He would then get up and walk around for 5 or 10 minutes and return to study for another 20 minutes. He had difficulty focusing on lectures, movies, or plays. During any task that required sustained attention, Luke Belden's mind tended to wander, or he would fall asleep because he put so much effort into concentrating. This pattern continued during his professional life, for example, even though his treatment of patients and recordkeeping in the office was in good order, his associates got the impression that he was haphazard in the way he organized things.

Dr. Belden did an internship at the University of Rochester at Strong Memorial Hospital and stayed on for three years to do a residency in psychiatry. Afterward, Belden accepted a two-year position at the National Institutes of Mental Health in Maryland, specializing in adolescent psychiatric treatment. He subsequently selected the small community of Appleton, Wisconsin, to begin his private practice in 1967. He wanted a small rural community, like the one in which he grew up, to raise his family and live.

He quickly settled into a busy private practice. However, his great energy and dedicated service to the community led him to take on additional responsibilities. For example, Belden was appointed an Examiner for the American Board of Psychiatry and Neurology, which certifies all psychiatrists and neurologists in the country. He was also a designated psychiatrist for the National Football League, working with Green Bay Packer players who had chemical dependency or mental health problems. Luke Belden also found time to work with a local community "free" clinic treating the homeless. In other words, Luke Belden was a high-profile physician with strong community ties and a high national standing and reputation.

During his second year of practice in Appleton at age 32, he experienced profound depression and sought psychiatric counseling. He had periodic episodes of suicidal thought involving a strong impulse to hang himself in the barn of his rural home. Indeed, he had a family history of depression and suicide. His father's paternal uncle, a pharmacist, had committed suicide in his mid-forties after attending an opera, and a paternal cousin committed suicide after graduating with honors from Carlton College. Luke Belden also had a nephew who was hospitalized for a year after a severe suicide attempt.

Three of his four sons were treated for depression, and two of them were diagnosed with ADHD. Luke Belden coped with this stress and illness by becoming an avid runner, exercising three to four miles daily. Exercising and keeping fit and taking antidepressant medications helped him cope with the depression.

When Luke Belden arrived in Appleton in 1967, he had four sons ages three months, three years, six years, and seven years old. In 1980, after 21 years of marriage, his wife Mary fell in love with a woman and left him and the children. They were divorced in 1982, and Luke Belden got full custody of the children. His ex-wife died of colon cancer in 1985. Belden did not remarry, which meant that Belden had sole responsibility for raising his sons. Dr. Belden also brought his two aged parents to live with his family when their health began to fail.

Dr. Belden's Medical Practice

When Dr. Belden arrived in Appleton, he joined a group of three psychiatrists called the Appleton Psychiatric Associates. This was a general psychiatric practice, and he was on call at St. Elizabeth's Hospital, which had the only psychiatric unit in the area. He took the hospital's psychiatric patients, including emergencies, day or night. He also covered as a general physician in the hospital's Emergency Department.

In 1984, the group broke up, and Allan Belden took a part-time position as the medical director of the psychiatric unit and continued his general psychiatric practice. He was also the medical director of a stress lab in the hospital known as the flotation tank. Dr. Belden became the psychiatric director of a small HMO in 1986 that entailed making hospital visits to see in-patients every day of the week except on his day off, Wednesday. He often stayed at the hospital till 9:00 P.M. and worked between 60 and 80 hours a week.

A Snitch Turns in Dr. Belden

Luke Belden's problems with the government began after he fired Joyce Sassman, a disgruntled 50-year-old billing clerk in his office. He hired her in 1984 through a temporary employment agency to fill in as a part-time receptionist and billing clerk. Sassman's communication skills were poor, and Dr. Belden finally fired Sassman in 1986 for being hostile to patients on the phone. She later found a job as a receptionist at Blue Cross Blue Shield (BCBS). While working at Blue Cross, she used the company's 1-800 fraud "hot line" to report that Dr. Belden was defrauding Blue Cross.

She told investigators that Dr. Belden was fraudulently billing the company for patients he did not treat. Almost 10 years later, Sassman's complaint was the core of the government's criminal prosecution of Luke Belden.

The Criminal Investigation Begins

Meridian Resource Corporation, a fraud investigation subsidiary of BCBS, launched an official investigation of Luke Belden in 1993. The investigation was carried out by Margaret Behrens, who worked at Blue Cross for 23 years. Her supervisor was Russell J. Streur, a 12-year employee of BCBS with 2 years of college education.

In October 1993, Streur ordered Behrens to identify all psychotherapists who billed Blue Cross for five or more "units" of treatment in a single day. A "unit" of treatment was one 45-minute session of psychotherapy per day. For example, if Dr. Belden billed Blue Cross for five units of psychotherapy, the company interpreted that to mean that he personally spent 45 minutes each with five patients. Behren explained the significance of this interpretation in trial testimony.

If (Belden) was billing (BCBS) for five or more units of psychotherapy in a day, (he) also did other things. There are only so many hours in a day. If they're billing us for this many (*units*), then they're billing other people.[27]

By examining the company's computerized billing record, they found that Dr. Belden billed Blue Cross for between 8 and 10 units per day. Using that unit measure of time, the company concluded that Belden would have had to provide between six and seven and a half hours of psychotherapy per day for the Blue Cross patients alone. Since Blue Cross only had a small share of the Appleton insurance market, they concluded that the number of Blue Cross bills submitted by Dr. Belden was suspiciously high. In other words, since Dr. Belden saw more non-Blue Cross patients than Blue Cross patients, the company surmised that Belden could not have treated as many Blue Cross patients as he claimed.

The next step in the company's investigation was to "flag" or suspend the processing of Dr. Belden's claims. This meant that the company's payments to Belden were stopped. His claims were sent to a fraud investigator who gathered together 105 claim forms submitted by Dr. Belden and contacted the patients by telephone. They found that 36 of the 105 patients said they had not actually seen Dr. Belden, despite the fact that the claims were billed in his name.

Behren asked the patients who had treated them. Some of the patients said they were treated by qualified therapists who worked in Dr. Belden's office. Other patients said they had been treated by Dr. Belden's nurses. This set off fraud alarm bells. Blue Cross's policy was not to pay for psychotherapy services performed by unlicensed nurses. Blue Cross paid only for psychotherapy performed by a psychiatrist or certified therapists with a Master's Degree and 3,000 hours of supervised therapy. In other words, Dr. Belden was not allowed to bill Blue Cross for psychotherapy services provided by his nurses.

In January 1994, Blue Cross sent the 105 claims to Dr. Belden's office and asked him to list the names of the persons who treated the patients. Belden's office manager placed the therapists' names on the claim forms and returned them. However, they did not list the names of the nurses who had treated the patients.

Blue Cross checked the names of the therapists on the claim forms against the names that patients said treated them. There were 10 claim forms with Dr. Belden's name on them but which patients said nurses had treated them. Blue Cross got statements from these patients confirming that they had been treated by nurses and not by Dr. Belden.

Blue Cross made no further attempt to contact Dr. Belden to reconcile the apparent discrepancy of the provider names on the claims. In fact, the only direct contact that Blue Cross made with Dr. Belden was in January 1994. Investigators told him to continue his billing practices and it would "get back to him." In 1995, Blue Cross removed the hold on Dr. Belden's insurance claims. Luke Belden interpreted that to mean that the company was satisfied with his billing claims. Indeed, Dr. Belden heard nothing more from Blue Cross until he was criminally indicted for fraud in 1999, more than five years later.

Coordinating Role of Appleton Police Department

After Blue Cross got advice from the Appleton District Attorney, it filed a complaint against Dr. Belden with the Appleton Police Department. Blue Cross fraud supervisor Russell Streur instructed Margaret Behrens to prepare a criminal case against Belden and wished her "good hunting."

The Blue Cross fraud investigator spoke with Officer Frank Groh of the Appleton Police Department even before the company had prepared the report alleging fraud by Luke Belden. The Appleton Police Department, in turn, contacted Mary Ducat, a fraud investigator for Employer's Health (now Humana) in April 1994. Groh asked if Humana had any billing concerns with Dr. Belden. After receiving the call, Ducat said she would look into it, and she made a series of calls of her own.

She called the Wisconsin Department of Health and Social Services and the state nurse licensing board to confirm that Belden's nurses were not qualified to provide psychotherapy to patients. She then called the OIG of HHS, the Postal Inspector, the District Attorney's Office, and the FBI to find out if they would be willing to investigate Dr. Belden for fraud. It was clear from the outset that Humana was searching for any law enforcement agency to launch a criminal investigation of Luke Belden.

Humana followed the same internal investigation that Blue Cross did. It placed a hold on Dr. Belden's claims and contacted his office to obtain the names of individuals who saw the patients. Humana sent out between 30 and 40 questionnaires to Dr. Belden's patients asking who had treated them. If they found claims with Dr. Belden's name on it but which the patients said nurses treated them, it was taken as evidence of criminal fraud. During May 1994, Humana sent a computer report containing the names and Social Security Numbers of 9,800 patients to Officer Groh to document Dr. Belden's fraudulent billing.

On May 31, 1994, Ducat sent a letter to Dr. Belden explaining that he was using the wrong CPT code to bill for patient treatment. He was using CPT 90844, individual therapy, for nurses' treatment of patients. Ducat said the that nurses were not qualified to provide psychotherapy to patients.

Dr. Belden responded to the letter by calling Ducat on June 3, 1994, asking what the proper CPT code was for nurses' treatment of patients. Ducat said that when nurses saw patients, Belden should bill the company for CPT 90862, which was a medication check. The individual psychotherapy CPT codes 90843 (30 minutes) and 90844 (45 minutes) were reserved for psychotherapy services provided only by psychiatrists or certified therapists, not nurses.

Dr. Belden explained that his nurses were under his direct supervision when they saw patients and that they did more than simply check patients' medications. Often, Dr. Belden would see the patients for the first 10 minutes with a nurse and have the nurse finish up the visit. Other times, the nurses would see the patient and then leave the examining room to get instructions from Dr. Belden and return to complete the visit.

Belden said that the nurses spent a lot of time going over with the patient their social, spiritual, and everyday activities. The nurses even knew how many cups of coffee or soft drinks a patient had in a day. It was a very thorough visit. Ducat responded that Humana would pay only for CPT code 90862 (medication check) when nurses saw patients. Dr. Belden reluctantly agreed to this and said that henceforth, he would bill the company for nurses' services using only CPT code 90862.

The significance of using CPT 90862 to Dr. Belden, however, was that he and many other psychiatrists regarded it as a "dirty" or unethical code. In fact, until Ducat instructed him to use CPT 90862 for nurses, he had refused to use that code. The reason is that the code was widely abused by large mental clinics, especially in major urban areas.

In these mental clinics, CPT 90862 was often used several times for the same patient in the process of checking various medications. It had no time limit. Luke Belden explained to his son that the code was "crazy," and was simply a way of "pumping" people through the system to make a lot of money.[28] He took pride in his work and wanted to provide quality service to his patients rather than making a lot of money.

FBI Undercover Operation

The FBI became involved in the investigation of Dr. Belden when Humana contacted them. On July 29, 1994, Ducat contacted Special Agent John Aziere, the FBI Agent in charge of the Milwaukee Division. The Milwaukee Division was responsible for 22 counties in northeastern Wisconsin, including Appleton. Ducat spoke to Aziere by phone and said that the Appleton Police Department had informed her that Dr. Belden may have defrauded Blue Cross and she suspected that Belden may have also defrauded Humana.

Agent Aziere went to Ducat's office and picked up a 134-page computer printout of patient information, including Social Security numbers, patient's first names, date of service, CPT codes, and the billing charges and amounts paid by Humana. Aziere also met with Detective Frank Groh at the Appleton Police Department and picked up similar computer files that Blue Cross sent to Groh's home. Neither the FBI nor the Appleton Police Department obtained court orders for these files. This is particularly egregious since many of Dr. Belden's patients were being treated for alcohol and drug addiction. Any disclosure of this information could ruin their careers and lives and is strictly forbidden by law.

After examining the billing claims and comparing the names on the forms with patient statements, Aziere apparently decided that the evidence was not strong enough to indict Dr. Belden. Instead of dropping the case, however, he decided to send in an undercover FBI agent to catch Dr. Belden in the act of fraudulently billing the companies.

Aziere assigned Agent George DeShazor (undercover name George DeShazer) to the case in late 1995. DeShazor was specially trained for the job. He had a bachelor's degree in psychology and sociology, a master's degree in clinical social work and was a practicing therapist in hospitals and outpatient clinics. DeShazor had even been in private practice himself. He later became an instructor at the FBI Academy in Quantico, Virginia, in the Behavioral Science Unit that focuses upon psychological crimes. He taught all new agents trained at the Academy in investigative psychology including police executives. He also consulted with law enforcement agencies throughout the country on detecting and combating psychological crimes.

In October 1995, while DeShazor was assigned to the Milwaukee Division, Agent Aziere asked DeShazor to become involved in the Belden investigation as an undercover agent. He undertook this undercover assignment without any prior experience or a subpoena from the USAO. Aziere told DeShazor of the allegations against Luke Belden. Most of DeShazor's prior undercover work involved sitting in a car as a decoy or performing a cameo role by sitting with someone who was posing as a dealer in a drug investigation or organized crime deal. This was the first time he was sent in as an undercover agent to investigate a physician.

DeShazor made an appointment with Dr. Belden using a false name, address, and phony mental illness. Correspondence between Dr. Belden's office and DeShazor was sent to the home address of Officer Groh from the Appleton Police Department and then forwarded to the prosecutors in the USAO and the FBI. When Agent DeShazor went for his appointments at Dr. Belden's office, Agent Aziere was present in Dr. Belden's parking lot, supervising DeShazor's visits.

During his appointments, DeShazor pretended that he was suffering from mild depression with symptoms of sleeplessness, loss of appetite, irritability, difficulty concentrating, and generally feeling low. DeShazor's job was to see whether he received a complete evaluation from Dr. Belden, or whether he was treated by nurses but billed for seeing Dr. Belden.

Agent DeShazor had his first appointment at Dr. Belden's office on October 30, 1995, and saw Luke Belden in his office alone. Belden spent about 30 minutes with DeShazor. Based upon follow-up questions to a questionnaire DeShazor filled out, Dr. Belden made an initial evaluation of dysphoric disorder or mild depression treatable with Prozac or Ambien.

Luke Belden recommended that DeShazor follow up this visit with a therapist in the office. The follow-up appointment lasted 50 minutes, and DeShazor described it as a "very good job." Agent DeShazor's third, and final, treatment at Dr. Belden's office involved seeing one of Dr. Belden's nurses for about 30 minutes. The nurse asked him about his symptoms and whether the medication was relieving them.

After about 15 minutes of questioning, the nurse left DeShazor to speak with Dr. Belden, who was in his office to verify whether the medication DeShazor was given was working or not. After this third visit, Agent DeShazor was taken off the case by his supervisor, Agent Aziere. In trial testimony, DeShazor was asked why he was taken off the case, and he said that he did not know. When he was asked whether he had enough knowledge of the case to decide to cease undercover work, he said no.[29]

Instead of dropping the case, however, the prosecutors decided to proceed with the investigation. In April 1996, between 10 and 15 armed agents from the FBI, OIG of Health and Human Services, and the State of Wisconsin raided Dr. Belden's office and seized hundreds of patient files, appointment books, and index cards that contained the handwritten notes of Belden's employees. They also downloaded Dr. Belden's computer, interviewed Luke Belden and the other staff members present in the office. Luke Belden asked repeatedly what they were doing wrong. The only answer he got was to keep on doing what he was doing. "We aren't saying you are doing anything wrong. Just keep on doing what you are doing."[30]

The agents were in the office from about 3:00 P.M. till 3:00 A.M. They had a search warrant and grand jury subpoenas for Dr. Belden's records. They said they needed the patients' files so that they could match patients' names with the names of the providers on the billing claims.

The Criminal Indictment of Luke Belden

On March 23, 1999, three years after the raid, Dr. Belden was charged with a 16-count federal indictment for defrauding private insurance companies from 1990 to 1996. The indictment was based upon Dr. Belden's claims for services provided to seven patients and FBI Special Agent George DeShazor working in an undercover capacity posing as a patient. The government interviewed almost 400 psychiatric patients in order to find five who would testify against Dr. Belden. The interviews reportedly began with an intimidating statement, "Did you know your doctor was a criminal?" During the trial, patients were not allowed to testify on Dr. Belden's behalf.

Luke Belden billed all but two of the appointments using CPT code 90844 (Individual Medical Psychotherapy by a physician for approximately 45–50 minutes). On the remaining two appointments, he submitted a bill using CPT code 90843 (Individual Medical Psychotherapy by a physician for approximately 20-30 minutes). All of the claims identified Luke Belden as the provider of service.

Four of the patients testified that their appointments had been with Dr. Belden's nurses. During trial testimony, Dr. Belden's nurses confirmed that fact, but said that they were not qualified to provide, nor did they provide, psychotherapy to patients. Special Agent DeShazor testified that at his third appointment on November 21, 1995 (which was billed as individual psychotherapy under CPT code 90843), he was treated by a nurse. The nurse testified that she saw DeShazor but did not provide psychotherapy to him.

The indictment alleged that Dr. Belden up-coded or overbilled for the length of patients' appointments. He routinely submitted claims to insurance companies indicating that patients had received individual psychotherapy for 40 to 50 minutes (CPT code 90844), when, in fact, they had only been treated for 30 minutes (CPT code 90843).

The government alleged that Dr. Belden concealed his "scheme to defraud" by directing his staff to submit claims to insurance companies using CPT codes 90843 and 90844, thereby, falsely billing the "victim" companies. The government claimed that Dr. Belden allowed his nurses to act as the primary caregivers for the majority of his patients and, thereby, fraudulently billed insurance companies for individual psychotherapy services.

Prosecutors argued that in order to conceal the fact that his nurses were providing psychotherapy, he ordered his staff not to sign or identify themselves on patients' progress notes. Dr. Belden, therefore, received payment for services that were not provided and for which he was not entitled. Luke Belden was also indicted for committing mail fraud because he used the U.S. mail to submit false bills to the insurance companies in a scheme to defraud them.

Failure to Prove Intent to Defraud

At the trial of Luke Belden, the government did not prove that his billing practices were wrong, much less that it was part of a scheme to defraud the insurance companies. This was made clear in the only expert testimony by Dr. Chester Schmidt, Jr., the Chairman of the Department of Psychiatry at Johns Hopkins University's Bay View Medical Center. Dr. Schmidt was also the Chair of the American Psychiatric Association's Work Group on Codes and Reimbursements and served on the American Medical Association's Relative Value Update Committee that sets the fee schedules for the Medicare program. He is also the author of two books on psychiatric coding. In other words, Schmidt helped create the psychiatric codes that the government used to indict Luke Belden.

Dr. Schmidt explained that the incidental psychotherapy services (the ones Luke Belden's nurses provided under his direct supervision) being provided by nurses was a widespread and accepted practice in psychiatry throughout the country. Given the vast experience of Belden's nurses and the degree of his supervision, the use of CPT Codes 90843 and 90844 (the psychotherapy codes) was, in fact, correct. Dr. Schmidt testified that the fees charged by Dr. Belden were "in the ballpark." He pointed out that even if Belden had used CPT Code 90862 (medication code), the flat rate he charged, that is to say between $100 and $110 for a half hour consultation, was reasonable. In fact, if Dr. Belden had used CPT 90862 instead, which had no time limit, he could have legitimately charged the insurance companies significantly more than he actually did using the psychotherapy codes. In other words, Belden did not use the billing codes for self-enrichment.

Furthermore, Schmidt said that Luke Belden did not hide the fact that he was using his nurses (called physician extenders) under his close supervision to treat patients. Throughout 1994, when Dr. Belden had direct contact with the insurance companies, he disclosed the fact that his nurses treated patients under his supervision.

Belden explained this to Blue Cross and Humana's fraud investigators Russell Streur and Mary Ducat. This was also explained to undercover FBI agent George DeShazor during his office visits. The office staff specifically informed DeShazor that Dr. Belden and his nurses billed jointly for their services at the rate of $100 per hour. In fact, Agent Deshazor signed a form acknowledging his payment for this service. Luke Belden also did not destroy or alter any of his billing records, and he did not instruct his staff to lie.

In addition, the billing system of the insurance companies was so chaotic and contradictory that it was virtually impossible for Dr. Belden to comply with all of their rules. Belden had to deal with six private insurance companies listed in the indictment. They were Blue Cross/Blue Shield, Wisconsin Physician Service, Guardian Life, American Medical Security, and Employers Health (now Humana). None of the companies gave Dr. Belden any instructions for billing, nor did they object to the claims he had been submitting to them for about 10 years.

In 1994, after Belden was contacted by Blue Cross, he asked their fraud supervisor, Russell Streur, how he should bill for nurses' supervised services. Streur said that "he didn't know." In fact, it was only at the end of 1994, when Mary Ducat of Humana contacted Dr. Belden, that Belden was told to submit claims for nurses' services under CPT code 90862 and he immediately complied with this request.

Despite these instructions, however, each insurance company had its own unpublished reimbursement policies. Blue Cross even had its own CPT billing codes. This meant that the companies reimbursed Dr. Belden for services provided by his nurses under different CPT codes.

The government's indictment assumed that Belden should have billed for nurses' services using CPT Code 90862. However, not all insurers named in the indictment reimbursed Dr. Belden for that code. Blue Cross and Humana reimbursed nurses under CPT code 90862; however, the Wisconsin Physician Service did not reimburse nurses under CPT code 90862. In other words, if Dr. Belden had billed Wisconsin Physician Services for nurses' services under 90862, he could have been indicted for fraudulent billing.

The prosecution's charge that Dr. Belden committed mail fraud is also without foundation. The definition of mail fraud is the use of U.S. mail for the purpose of committing a criminal act or as "part of a scheme to defraud." This requires that the government prove that Dr. Belden fraudulently submitted claims to the insurance companies. There is no evidence of this, however.

The insurance companies did not provide any written instructions to doctors for submitting reimbursement claims. The only claim form that was used by physicians was the Health Care Financing Administration (HCFA, now CMS) 1500 form. It is used throughout the medical industry for reimbursement from Medicare and private insurance companies.

The HCFA 1500 form clearly states that a physician may bill for services "incident to a physicians' professional service if that service is under the doctor's immediate supervision although an incidental part of a physician's service, is furnished in a physician's office and the services of non-physicians are included on the physician's bills."

Dr. Belden's bills met all of the conditions set forth by the government. If a private insurance company had additional conditions for billing, it must provide written guidance or instructions as to the proper billing procedures. None of the companies did so.

The Judge's Verdict

The presiding federal judge, Rudolph T. Randa, refused to allow the only expert witness, Dr. Chester Schmidt, Jr., to testify till six weeks after the initial trial and then required that his testimony be in writing. Even after Schmidt's testimony was accepted, the judge dismissed it by stating that Dr. Belden would have to rely upon evidence other than Dr. Schmidt's to demonstrate the absence of "fraudulent intent."[31] However, Since Dr. Belden's alleged fraud was based upon his use of CPT billing codes, and since Dr. Schmidt is the foremost expert on psychiatric CPT codes, this is tantamount to dismissing the only evidence that could convict or exonerate Luke Belden. The American judicial system had been turned on its head. Dr. Belden had to prove his innocence rather than the state's proving him guilty beyond a reasonable doubt.

Dr. Belden opted for a court trial presided over by a U.S. District Judge Randa in the mistaken belief that a judge, rather than a jury, would be fairer and better able to understand the complex coding issues of the case. To everyone's surprise, after the trial ended, Judge Randa delayed making a decision for one year and then handed down a stunning verdict of guilty on all counts.

The judge said that despite the absence of financial gain, Luke Belden knew that he was using the wrong CPT codes to bill, and he intentionally used the U.S. mail to carry out a scheme to defraud the insurance companies. Judge Randa entirely misconstrued Dr. Belden's answer to a single question during cross examination to arrive at that judgment. The question was, "Now, you know now, do you not, that wrong codes were being used?" Luke Belden's response was, "Yes, I realize now."[32] However, Dr. Belden was simply responding to the billing instructions he received from Mary Ducat of Humana in 1994. Furthermore, Dr. Schmidt contradicted Luke Belden's statement during his testimony by saying that the codes Dr. Belden used to bill the companies were, in fact, correct. Nevertheless, Judge Randa ignored Dr. Schmidt's testimony and focused upon what he described as Dr. Belden's so-called admission of guilt.

The government's case against Dr. Belden was based upon a complete misunderstanding of the practice of psychiatry and the use of CPT codes for reimbursement. It created a legal precedent that dramatically expanded the criminal prosecutions of physicians. It gives insurance companies the power to create crimes in order to limit and recover payments made to doctors for services rendered to patients. In other words, it criminalizes private medical reimbursement practices.

The Impact on Dr. Belden and Family

The impact of the trial upon Luke Belden and his family has been devastating. His mental state visibly deteriorated during the ordeal. By the spring of 1999, he suffered from major depression, and by the summer of 1999, he was diagnosed with bipolar disorder, by the time of the hearing, Dr. Belden was obsessional. His mental state continued to decline and began to show signs of dementia. Dr. Belden was unable to manage his financial affairs, and he exhibited bizarre behavior.

This behavior included such things as attempting to go shopping wearing nothing but mosquito netting, carpeting the bottom of a pond near his home in order to smooth out the bottom, urinating in the corner of a room at night, and applying sandpaper to rust spots on his Lexus automobile, thus damaging the finish of the car.

The cost of his legal defense exceeded $1.1 million. After the trial, he was ordered to pay $125,000 in restitution to the insurance companies and spent three months in a federal prison for psychiatric evaluation and was given one-year supervised probation. He was ordered to surrender his medical license and thus is unable to fulfill his lifelong calling of healing the sick and lame. Indeed, he wished to treat veterans returning from Iraq who were suffering the effects of head trauma for which he had specialized expertise.

Dr. Belden now lives in a 100-year-old family farmhouse with four bedrooms and one and one half baths with average furniture. The residence is on 120 acres of land, which was used as a tree farm for future harvest. Allan Belden originally willed the land to the Nature Conservancy but since two-thirds of his retirement savings was wiped out by his legal defense, he reluctantly decided to divide it and will it to his sons.

After Belden's indictment in 1999, he had a compulsion to commit suicide. He had a recurring impulse to hang himself in his barn and was on 24-hour suicide watch. Two weeks after the verdict, Sande Krizek, Allan Belden's psychiatric nurse, fiancée, and constant companion for seven years, called his son, Stuart, crying and reported that Luke said he was going to the barn and "shoot his brains out" as everyone would be better off. Since 2001, however, with the help of Sande, therapy, and medication, he has regained his mental stability.

Belden lost 20 to 25 pounds during the ordeal and slept only about two hours at night. He took numerous medications to control his psychiatric symptoms. These included Wellbutrin and Prozac for depression, Adderall for attention deficit, and Periactin and Clonazapam for sleep.

Belden's son, Stuart Belden, described his father as his best friend and said that Luke Belden aged by 10 years during his trial. Stuart Belden even blamed his divorce and failure in his real estate career on the stress of taking care of his father's legal defense.

Patsy Vargo and Allan Belden are struggling to cope with an inexplicable and unjust criminal indictment and prosecution. They are extremely dedicated physicians who served the sick and disadvantaged of their communities. Their prosecution by the government establishes a horrific precedent for all physicians.

5

JUDICIAL PREJUDICE, STATE TERRORISM, AND FORCED MEDICATION: THE CASES OF JEFFREY J. RUTGARD, M.D., GEORGE O. KRIZEK, M.D., AND CHARLES T. SELL, D.D.S.

The prosecution of Jeffrey Rutgard, George Krizek, and Charles Sell provide insight into the egregious and destructive nature of the government's law enforcement policy targeting doctors for alleged fraud. The Rutgard and Krizek cases illustrate the government's malicious use of ambiguous billing codes to prosecute physicians and the Sell case involves the imprisonment of a dentist without trial based upon fraud charges.

JEFFREY J. RUTGARD, M.D.

Dr. Jeffrey Jay Rutgard was a prominent 40-year-old married San Diego ophthalmologist with four children, ages one through five, when he became a victim of the government's war on doctors. Without warning, at 6:00 A.M. on April 27, 1992, his home and offices were raided by armed federal and state agents wearing FBI and police jackets. The media were tipped off in advance of the raid and were present at Dr. Rutgard's offices photographing and interviewing patients, agents, and employees.

The raid was widely reported on TV, radio, and in the newspapers. News of the raid was aired on the local TV station Channel 10 the same day at 5:00 P.M. San Diego television news reported that "all medical records were seized from prominent La Jolla ophthalmological surgeon Dr. Jeffrey Jay Rutgard." The day after the raid, the newspapers reported a statement by Sanford Feldman, deputy state attorney general, working with the Medical Board of California (MBC), to the effect that the board would immediately seek to suspend Dr. Rutgard's medical license.[1] This statement was made before the medical board met to consider the case and before Dr. Rutgard had an opportunity to defend himself against the accusation. State Attorney General Lazar elaborated by saying that "Dr. Rutgard violated about every medical ethic you can imagine."[2]

Jeff Rutgard's medical license was suspended on May 15, 1992, more than a year before Dr. Rutgard's case was heard by an administrative law judge of the California Medical Board. Before the raid, Jeff Rutgard was never even told that there were any complaints against him nor was he given an opportunity to respond to the complaints. He had no reason even to suspect that he was under investigation.

During his 12 years of medical practice involving more than 22,000 patients and 10,000 surgeries there were no mortalities nor did any patients lose their vision. He had only one malpractice suit, and the judge in that case dismissed it. Furthermore, every review (126 since the end of 1991) of his patient charts including the medical and surgical records of 50-150 patients by the California Medical Review, Inc. (Medicare's auditor of doctors' billing in California) for medical necessity was approved. In other words, Jeff Rutgard had a peerless record.

The Office of Inspector General (OIG) removed more than 22,000 documents and patient files from his home and offices. The patients who were present in the offices were photographed and questioned about the need for their surgeries, and some were taken to competing doctors nearby for second opinions.

Employees were told to go home and seek employment elsewhere. Agents placed signs on the office doors informing patients to seek eye care somewhere else. Dr. Rutgard was prevented from entering his own offices from Monday through Saturday, 6:00 A.M. to 6:00 P.M. He was not allowed to display his name at his office buildings, and the government never returned his medical records, office equipment, or patient files.

After numerous requests from Dr. Rutgard's attorney, in July 1992, the OIG finally allowed one of his employees to go to the OIG's office two days a week for three hours a day to copy patients' records and billings which had been removed from his offices by government agents during the raid. Defense attorneys were unable to keep up with the government's constant changing of patients named in the accusations.

At various time, prior to the court hearings, both the medical board prosecutor and the federal prosecutor would release thousands of pages of documents all at once. Defense attorneys did not have enough time to copy and respond to the medical records in question. Without copies of the patients' records the defense was at a disadvantage. It was impossible for Rutgard's attorney to respond to the government's accusations at the medical board hearing.

The MBC also took the highly unusual step of invoking the most drastic suspension possible of Dr. Rutgard's medical license. It used the Presley Bill (SB 2375) that took effect in January 1991. The bill empowered the board to suspend the license of any physician who represented an "immediate danger" to the public.

The legislation was designed for use only in the most extreme circumstances, involving doctors who were alcoholics, drug addicts, or who sexually abused, killed, or maimed their patients. Clearly, this did not apply to Jeff Rutgard. During the 12 years of his practice, Dr. Rutgard never blinded or killed a patient. Nevertheless, the deputy state attorney general, Sanford

Feldman, insisted that the board make the most drastic suspension possible of Dr. Rutgard's license.

Two and a half years later, in October 1994, Dr. Rutgard was tried in a federal court and convicted of defrauding the government of $65,140.02 for "unnecessary surgery" and was ordered to pay $16.2 million in restitution. The government also took away his medical license, his practice, his family savings, his home and sentenced him to more than 11 years in federal prison. In order to understand the government's prosecution of Dr. Rutgard, it is necessary to examine the trap that the federal and state governments set to ensnare him.

The Federal Prosecutorial Trap

In 1989, Richard Kusserow, the inspector general (IG) of the OIG, targeted high-volume eye doctors for fraud investigation. OIG investigators started to look for high-profile scapegoats to blame for rising Medicare costs. Kusserow focused upon the explosive growth in ophthalmologists' ambulatory surgical centers (ASCs), which increased by 300 percent from 1984 to 1989.

Increasing numbers of Medicare beneficiaries age 65 or more were having eye surgeries to remove cataracts, and they were going to eye surgical centers instead of hospitals. The surgical centers were not only more comfortable for patients, but they were safer, freer of hospital infection, and they saved the government and patients money. Unlike hospital patients, surgical center patients did not have to disrobe, wear open gowns, or be cold. They were given a clean smock to wear over their clothes. Surgical center patients do not have to wait in long lines with other hospital patients who are agonizing in pain over gallbladder, prostate surgery, hysterectomies, or emergency surgeries. They are not exposed to hospital infections and therefore patients experienced few eye infections, although thousands of surgeries are performed. Patients are in and out of the surgical centers within an hour and are back playing golf, driving, or at work the same day.

Surgical centers also saved Medicare money. For example, the local hospital near Dr. Rutgard's practice, Scripps Memorial Hospital, was paid between $4,000 and $5,000 per eye surgery for the use of the hospital operating room. This did not include the fee paid to the surgeon or the anesthesiologist. Medicare paid a hospital between $7,000 to $10,000 plus $500 to $1,200 to the hospital anesthesiologist plus a surgeon's fee of $2,200.

By contrast, Dr. Rutgard's Medicare approved surgery center received $1,000 for every cataract surgery performed. Rutgard received about $700 from Medicare for each cataract surgery (80 percent of the Medicare-allowed $900 reimbursement). His anesthesiologist received between $100 and $150 dollars per eye surgery. This represented a savings of about $5,900 for each cataract surgery.

Therefore, if Scripps Hospital performed over 1,000 cataracts per year from 1987 through 1992 and if we take half of the savings from Rutgard's surgery of $2,850 times 1,000 cataracts per year times six years, the savings to

Medicare would be $17 million. This is the reason that Medicare preferred to have eye surgeries performed in high-volume surgical centers like Dr. Rutgard's instead of at hospitals.

Because of their safety, convenience, and savings, the number of eye surgeries in surgery centers grew rapidly. Indeed, cataract surgeries became the most popular surgery among seniors. By 1991, an estimated 45 percent of the roughly 30 million Medicare beneficiaries received eye surgery that was paid for by Medicare. The most common eye disease was cataract, representing about 41 percent of patient treatment and 1.2 million surgeries. The cost of this was more than 12 percent of Medicare's entire budget. Kusserow felt that the growth in the cost of eye surgeries had to be controlled.

To carry out this mission, Kusserow targeted 84 high-volume ophthalmologists throughout the country. These were eye doctors who received more than $1 million from Medicare in 1987. He did this ostensibly to determine if their operations were "medically necessary." Based upon the survey, the OIG concluded that "high-volume ophthalmologists are more likely to provide medically unnecessary services."[3]

The Health Care Financing Administration (HCFA) strongly disagreed with this conclusion, however. HCFA said that "we do not believe that high-volume ophthalmologists are more likely to provide medically unnecessary services, high volume does not equate to overutilization." HCFA went on to say that cataract surgery is already subject to the "most intensive review" *before* being approved for Medicare payment.[4]

Kusserow rejected HCFA's advice and said that the agency should intensify its monitoring of high-volume ophthalmologists. It is clear that what was driving Kusserow was the burgeoning growth in Medicare payments for the removal of seniors' cataracts. Since Kusserow had already claimed that 10 percent of total government health expenditure was due to fraud, by his own logic, he was obliged to find 10 percent fraud in Medicare payments to eye doctors.

Since high-volume eye doctors received the largest payments from Medicare, and since there were only a few hundred of them, they were easy targets. The OIG also felt that if they prosecuted high-profile ophthalmologists, it would discourage eye doctors from performing cataract surgeries and would slow the growth in Medicare costs for eye surgeries. Indeed, after Dr. Rutgard was prosecuted, there was a reported decline of between 5 and 10 percent in Medicare bills for eye surgeries.

State Prosecutorial Trap

In 1991, the MBC was in the throes of a political crisis. The board was responsible for licensing and disciplining doctors for unprofessional conduct. Allegations of doctors' misconduct were investigated by the MBC and were turned over to the state Attorney General's Office for prosecution.

A political crisis erupted in the MBC after the publication of two reports. The first was released in 1989 called "Physician Discipline in California: A

Code Blue Emergency." It was sponsored by Robert Fellmeth's Center for Public Interest Law at the University of San Diego. The report concluded that the MBC was underfunded, was slow to respond to patient complaints, and had a huge backlog of cases it had not investigated.

This was followed by a devastating second report prepared by the California Highway Patrol (CHP) and released in 1991. The California Department of Consumer Affairs asked CHP to investigate "serious allegations of misconduct" by the Enforcement Unit of the MBC. In asking the CHP to investigate the MBC, the director said that "misconduct may have jeopardized the health, safety and welfare of hundreds of California citizens."[5]

CHP was asked to investigate the medical board instead of the Attorney General's office because of a potential conflict of interest between the Attorney General, Dan Lungren, and his father Dr. John Lungren, who was on the medical board.

The CHP report alleged that the medical board was guilty of shredding files and "case dumping" or the unwarranted closing of complaints against physicians without any investigation. The board also had a huge backlog of about 1,200 cases awaiting adjudication, including 350 cases that had not even been filed.

The report highlighted shoddy MBC investigation of five patient deaths in 1989 at Los Angeles' Martin Luther King, Jr. Hospital. One of the deaths involved a car crash in which an accident victim sustained fractured ribs and a lacerated liver. The physician at the emergency room overlooked the injuries, prescribed a painkiller, and sent the patient home. Twelve hours later, the patient returned to the hospital and died. The medical board closed the case without referring it for discipline.

Release of the CHP report set off a firestorm of public outrage against the medical board. In response to public indignation, state Senator Robert Presley introduced Senate Bill 2375 to create a special physician discipline system and transfer individual cases to an administrative law judge panel.

The significance of the new discipline system was that it made it easier to get convictions of doctors. There were three major changes. The first was that hearsay evidence was acceptable in administrative law cases rather than proof "beyond a reasonable doubt" as required in court trials. The second is that unlike court trials, statutes of limitation do not apply in administrative law cases. Hence, cases that were more than five years old could be heard by administrative law panels.

A third change in the physician discipline regime was the passage of a new administrative law called the Business and Professions Code (Section 125.3). This law empowered the medical board to recover the cost of investigation and prosecution from convicted physicians. It gave the California Medical Board a financial incentive to prosecute doctors. Such "cost-sharing" laws represent a significant threat to the constitutional due process rights of physicians. Dr. Rutgard's medical license was suspended under the authority of the Presley bill, and he was one of the first physicians to be tried by an administrative law judge.

The political fallout stemming from the Fellmeth and CHP reports was far-reaching. A new president of the medical board was appointed along with six new board members, and a new executive director was selected. Before 1990, the MBC's primary mission was physician rehabilitation, emphasizing the education of doctors about clinical practices and billing procedures.

After 1992, the mission shifted to investigation and prosecution. In the board's new law-enforcement role, there was the danger that it would overreact to sensationalized media reports of lack of physician discipline. Public pressure to discipline and prosecute bad doctors created the potential for abuse.

Faced with mounting criticism that the medical board was not doing enough to protect the public from incompetent and dangerous physicians, the board promised to increase the number of physician investigations dramatically (from 264 in 1992 to 600 in 1993). Indeed, more than 70 percent of the board's 1991–1992 budget was devoted to law enforcement.

The MBC was pressured to produce statistical proof that it was serving the public interest. A Public Citizen report in 1992 claimed that the MBC "was still not doing enough," and it ranked California 37th in the country for physician discipline.[6] In 1991, California reported 230 disciplinary actions against physicians, which averaged 2.94 actions per 1,000 doctors. This compared to the national average of 5.19 actions. According to the report, the medical board was not doing enough to discipline doctors. The report recommended that the board use looser standards of evidence to "improve its performance."

Representatives of the MBC tried to defend the board by saying that other states included dentists, chiropractors, and massage therapists in their discipline numbers. Nevertheless, the MBC came under intense public pressure to produce proof that it was severely disciplining physicians. The sensationalized media coverage of this issue created a hysterical atmosphere that distorted public perceptions. The MBC's effort to satisfy public demands led to the unjust punishment of many physicians.

Paul Pfingst, the San Diego district attorney, even acknowledged the destructive impact of the MBC's increased policing powers upon the lives and careers of physicians. He said that "a lifetime of service should not be at risk because of a single accusation."[7] He said that the MBC's current approach is like "using a cannon to kill a mosquito."

Richard Turner, a Sacramento attorney, explained the danger of overkill and said that "sometimes you just need to retrain doctors, give them a 'dutch uncle' talk. This is a lot cheaper and more effective in the long run than a full-blown prosecution."[8]

In response to the MBC's growing police powers, Robert Bowden, M.D., an Encinitas cardiologist, founded an organization called Physicians Opposed to Scurrilous and Scandalous Enforcement (POSSE). He organized POSSE to help protect doctors from unjust accusations by the medical board. Dr. Bowden explained the circumstances that led to the decision to form POSSE. Bowden received a late-night call from a friend and a physician who urgently wanted to speak to him at his home. When Dr. Bowden arrived, he found his friend agonizing over whether to sign an admission of guilt the next day in a MBC case. The doctor had already spent about $40,000 in legal fees defending himself after an undercover agent tricked him into prescribing a narcotic.

At five o'clock the next morning, Dr. Bowden received another call but this time it was from the emergency room of the hospital where his friend was experiencing chest pains. Dr. Bowden said, "I was really angry because they not only destroyed the livelihood of a good friend of mine, but they also almost killed him out of stress."[9]

A Brilliant Eye Surgeon

In 1981, Dr. Rutgard began his practice in San Diego, California. Initially, he worked in the medical practice of Dr. Amos Root. Rutgard purchased Dr. Root's practice in September 1982 when Root became ill and needed a replacement. Jeff Rutgard took care of Dr. Root's patients when he was out of town the previous year. Dr. Root was very pleased with Dr. Rutgard's treatment of his patients and picked him over others to take over his practice.

In 1986, Dr. Rutgard was chosen by Dr. John Bikerton, the oldest practicing ophthalmologist in La Jolla, to take over his practice. Jeff Rutgard was chosen over other eye doctors who had offices in La Jolla and also wanted to purchase Bikerton's practice. These physicians included Dr. Max Smith, who had worked with Dr. Bikerton for 10 years assisting him in surgery and Dr. Barry Kassar. Both doctors competed with Dr. Rutgard for patients and became expert prosecution witnesses against Jeff Rutgard at his trial.

In 1989, Rutgard opened up a modern high-tech eye surgery center in La Jolla, California, called the La Jolla Eye Surgery Center. The eye center took four years to plan, two years to build, and it cost over six million dollars. The center had 10 fully equipped exam rooms and 2 operating rooms. He had a staff of about 35 employees, 5 of whom were highly trained and certified ophthalmic technicians, expert in refraction, glaucoma tonometry, visual field test, fundus photos, and assisting in surgery. With his efficient organization and expert staff he was able to examine between 100 and 130 patients a day. About 80 percent of his patients were Medicare beneficiaries. He treated 22,000 patients from 1988 to April 1992 when his practice was shut down. During that period, Dr. Rutgard received $15 million from the government for patients' treatment. This is not unusual for high-volume eye doctors.

Dr. Rutgard's practice grew as his outstanding surgical skills were spread by word of mouth. He kept an exhausting schedule, working $6^1/_2$ days a week, 16 hours a day. He also made trips to medical meetings and did not take vacations. His surgical skills were so widely recognized that other ophthalmologists sent their family members to him for treatment. Dr. Rutgard was one of the highest-volume cataract surgeons in the country, performing over 1,000 cataract operations a year. He performed most operations at his eye surgery center in La Jolla.

In order to understand the rapid expansion and success of Dr. Rutgard's practice, it is necessary to be aware of the revolution in cataract surgery that occurred at the time he started his practice. Until the 1980s, most eye surgeons used the intracapsular method of removing cataracts (the lens is removed along with its surrounding capsule or envelope). It requires between 6 and 12 stitches per eye.

Since that time, a revolutionary new surgical technique was developed for the removal of cataracts called extra capsular phacoemulsification or "phaco" for short. Phaco surgery involves the use of a sound wave instrument and requires none or only one stitch. It is now regarded as the ultimate in modern surgical technology. Of the roughly 300 eye surgeons in the San Diego area in 1991, Dr. Rutgard was the only one who performed "no-stitch phaco" cataract surgery. His competitors were performing intracapsular surgery.

The chief advantage of phaco surgery is that it requires a very small incision (3 millimeters) takes less time, there is less trauma to the eye, and there are fewer complications. The large incision intracapsular method involves more bleeding, has a much slower recovery time, and the results are not as good. To perform the small incision phaco method properly, a surgeon must be skilled in microsurgery as well as having performed a significant number of phaco surgeries on a frequent basis As a result of his experience and skill, Dr. Rutgard had a significantly smaller number of complications compared to most other eye surgeons.

It is not a procedure for doctors who do not perform surgeries on a regular basis. Learning how to perform the phaco surgical method is exacting and difficult. Thus in the early 1980s, fewer than 2 percent of the eye surgeons in the country had the necessary skills to perform phaco surgery. Indeed, the procedure must be done with great care and precision and is only as good as the surgeon's skills. Everyone, including the judge in Dr. Rutgard's trial, acknowledged that Dr. Rutgard was a "great surgeon." According to the American Academy of Ophthalmology, risk of visual loss due to cataract surgery is less than 5 percent for all eye doctors (using both the intracapsular and phaco methods). Dr. Rutgard's practice had a visual risk of less than 1 percent.

There were approximately 17,000 ophthalmologists in the country at the time who performed cataract extractions. However, the number of operations by eye doctors varied greatly. For example, some doctors performed between 5 and 10 surgeries per year, whereas the busiest cataract surgeons such as Jeffrey Rutgard performed a thousand or more operations a year. Dr. Rutgard was among fewer than 200 ocular high-volume eye doctors in the country at the time. He was a member of the Society for Excellence in Eyecare (SEE), which included the top 40 ophthalmologists in the country.

Like all high-volume ophthalmologists, Rutgard had a community relations program in which his staff visited senior citizens centers and nursing and retirement homes on a regular basis and provided free screening tests for cataract and eyelid problems. He also sent vans to the senior centers to bring patients to his clinics for further examination.

The Conspiracy against Dr. Rutgard

The conspiracy against Dr. Rutgard originated with three disgruntled ex-employees. They were George Butera, Jean Havel, and Shirley Duncan. Butera was Dr. Rutgard's office manager, Jean Havel was his billing clerk and Butera's reputed lover, and Shirley Duncan was a surgical assistant. Butera had worked with Havel before joining Dr. Rutgard's practice and brought her with him when he was hired. After Butera and Duncan were fired by Dr. Rutgard in October 1991, the three of them carried out a scheme to report Dr. Rutgard to state and federal law enforcement agencies in order to collect money as whistleblowers.

In sworn testimony and declarations, Shirley Duncan's brother, Thomas Glen Thomas, and her ex-husband, Glen Duncan, described the nature of the conspiracy. Thomas G. Thomas made the following statement at the MBC hearing on January 20, 1993:

> My sister (Shirley Duncan) was unhappy. She didn't feel like she was being treated properly in the office. She said that she and George (Butera) were altering charts. She probably could write anything on the charts, and Jeff (Rutgard) would sign them because Dr. Rutgard trusted her so much. She was falsifying charts, and George were going to submit these to insurance companies or Medicare. They planned to scam some money. It was going to make them rich.[10]

Shirley Duncan's ex-husband, Glen C. Duncan gave the following sworn declaration on January 1, 1997, in San Diego:

> I have always thought that Shirley called the Feds. She jumped at the chance to talk to the Feds—probably mostly to feel important. She was on "Nightline" and thought she was going to get money from "Inside Edition." Shirley brought original patient charts home. She took notes from the charts to get her story straight and would then call the others to tell them how it was. The three main players were Jean Havel, Shirley, and George Butera. They didn't get greedy until they thought they could get money from Dr. Rutgard on the malicious prosecution case. They collaborated greatly to make sure this would stick against Dr. Rutgard.[11]

On the date that Dr. Rutgard fired Jean Havel in October 1991 (one day after Butera was fired), Havel made the following threat in the presence of Carman Chavez, Havel's supervisor in the billing department.[12] Havel stated, "This is the beginning of a little earthquake, Carmen. Many people are going to leave and people like yourself will stay, but this is only the beginning."

The fired employees made good this threat and reported Jeff Rutgard to the medical board and to the OIG of Health and Human Services (HHS) for alleged fraud. Before doing so, they received assurances from the federal government that they would not be investigated for fraud. This encouraged them to proceed with their conspiracy against Dr. Rutgard.

Denying Rutgard's Due Process of the Law

In the medical board and OIG's eagerness to suspend Dr. Rutgard's medical license and criminally indict him for fraud, they egregiously violated Dr. Rutgard's due process rights. Deputy Attorney General Sanford Feldman and medical board investigators Gerald O'Donnell, Tracy Hutchinson, and Cynthia Brandenburg were determined to prove that Jeff Rutgard was guilty of "gross negligence and incompetence."

In order to do this, they followed a three-fold strategy. They used the perjured testimony of Dr. Rutgard's ex-employees, they solicited complaints from a handful of former patients, and used local, competing doctors to testify against Jeff Rutgard.

The MBC's Use of Perjured Testimony

The discrepancy in the testimony of the ex-employees at the medical board hearing, at Rutgard's criminal trial, and their testimony in 1997, at Rutgard's federal appeals case, reveals the extent of their perjury. The medical board accepted their hearsay evidence without question, however. For example, in Butera's testimony on December 21, 1993, he made the following accusation against Dr. Rutgard.[13] He said that Rutgard routinely took files home to alter patients' diagnoses fraudulently in order to justify unnecessary operations. Butera also claimed that Dr. Rutgard falsified eye test results and up-coded patient treatment to justify unnecessary surgeries. Butera claimed that Rutgard fraudulently falsified photographs of patients to justify eye lid surgeries. The other ex-employees corroborated Butera's testimony. For example, Shirley Duncan, the former surgical assistant, testified that Jeff Rutgard billed Medicare for surgeries that he did not perform.

On cross-examination by Dr. Rutgard's lawyer on April 1, 1997, Butera contradicted his earlier testimony.[14] Butera responded to the following questions.

> Q. During the years that you worked for Dr. Rutgard, did he ever tell you personally to submit a fraudulent bill to Medicare?
> A. No.
> Q. Do you have any personal knowledge that Dr. Rutgard's examinations were done fraudulently, illegally, improperly?
> A. No.
> Q. Do you have any personal knowledge that the examinations and/or surgeries that he performed did not in fact match the billing that was sent to Medicare?
> A. No, I wasn't in the operating room. I wasn't in the exam room, so no.

Likewise, on cross-examination, the other ex-employees contradicted their earlier, perjured testimony. For example, in 1996, Shirley Duncan admitted that she was not present when Dr. Rutgard examined patients and therefore could not say what actually happened.[15]

The Medical Board Breaks the Law

The MBC violated its own laws in order to manufacture evidence of Dr. Rutgard's negligence and incompetence. According to the "Guidebook to the Laws Governing the Practice of Medicine by Physicians and Surgeons" published by the State of California Department of Consumer Affairs Board of Medical Quality Assurance in 1992, the MBC may only investigate complaints against physicians after patients contact their doctor and submit a complaint in writing to the medical board (Business and Professions Code, Section 800). Furthermore, MBC investigators may lawfully have access only to the records of patients who have filed complaints against their doctors.

Totally disregarding these laws, MBC investigators scoured thousands of Dr. Rutgard's patient files without permission to identify potential complainants. Nevertheless, after going through 22,000 confidential patient records, investigators were only able to identify 30 patients whom they hoped might submit formal complaints against Dr. Rutgard. The investigators proceeded to harass these mostly elderly patients to sign MBC documents accusing Dr. Rutgard of negligence or dishonesty. For example, Harold Diaz made the following declaration on December 30, 1992.

> I am a very satisfied patient of Dr. Jeffrey Rutgard. I resent that Investigator (*Gerald*) O'Donnell from the California Medical Board has phoned me several times trying to coerce me into testifying against Dr. Rutgard. I am tired of his many phone calls, and I consider this to be harassment.[16]

Some of Dr. Rutgard's patients, such as Armando Gabriana, inadvertently signed a complaint against Jeff Rutgard when it was handed to him, but later recanted the statement. On March 17, 1993, Gabriana attested to this:

> The declaration that I was presented with was written by Gerald O'Donnell, and I do not feel comfortable with signing a declaration for the Medical Board that I did not write. I was contacted by the Medical Board and persuaded to get involved. I am choosing to remove myself and my records from this case.[17]

Some patients, such a Virgina Robinson, were pressured by MBC investigators to see other eye doctors in order to concoct expert medical testimony against Dr. Rutgard. On December 17, 1992, Robinson made the following declaration:

> After Dr. Jeffrey's office was raided, I received a phone call from an agent (*of the medical board*) who wanted to see me. Two men came to my house and asked

me questions about Dr. Rutgard. Soon afterward, I received a phone call from someone from the same office called Tracy (Hutchinson). She asked if she could come over and take me for a second opinion on my eyes. She phoned me two more times, so I finally went. Tracy took me to La Jolla to see two doctors in the same office. One doctor asked me if I really thought I had cataracts. That was a silly question. Dr. Rutgard takes care of people so well. I don't know why anyone would want to do this to him. I know it must be jealous doctors because so many patients go to him and love him.[18]

Competing Doctors Join the Conspiracy

MBC investigators recruited local doctors in the San Diego area who were in competition with Jeff Rutgard to testify in support of revoking his medical license and prosecute him for fraud. This is a clear violation of the laws governing the medical board. According to the MBC Task Force on Medical Quality Review, medical experts who consider complaints against a physician must be in the doctor's own specialty and practice in a "geographic area different from the respondent so as to avoid any appearance of conflict."[19] This is usually interpreted to be 500 miles from the locale of the physician being investigated. Contrary to the rule, the government used local eye doctors within a radius of about five miles of Dr. Rutgard's practice. Not only were these doctors in direct competition with Rutgard, but they were not even qualified to evaluate his practice. Most of them did not do the "no-stitch" cataract surgery in which Rutgard specialized. The doctors who testified against Dr. Rutgard primarily performed the older, large-incision cataract surgery.

Furthermore, nationally renowned experts, Dr. Henry Baylis, Dr. Dennis Shepard, Dr. John Corboy, and Dr. E. Lee Rice, not only contradicted these witnesses but accused the doctors of a "conspiracy." For example, Dr. Henry Baylis, the Chief of Ophthalmic Surgery at UCLA for 15 years, made the following statement:

> In reviewing the charts of Dr. Jeff Rutgard reviewed by Drs. Art Perry, Stephen Pratt and Lee Nordan, I see a conspiracy among the three doctors. They are associated with each other and are in league to stop this worthy physician from practicing medicine. I fail to see how a medical board can pick the direct competitors of a physician to judge him.[20]

Dr. E. Lee Rice, a professor at the University of California, San Diego School of Family Medicine and Pediatrics Medicine, concurred with Dr. Baylis' opinion:

> Dr. Rutgard has been the subject of a biased and prejudicial investigation. It involved deceit, trickery, lies and supposed expert opinions from competitive physicians with an inherent conflict of interest.[21]

Dr. John Corboy, a Clinical Associate Professor of Surgery at the University of Hawaii, explained the biased nature of the government's medical witnesses. He said the claim that Jeff Rutgard performed "unnecessary surgery" is bogus. Cataracts all get worse daily. There are merely degrees of necessity for the surgery.

For the best results and safety of patients, the new "no-stitch" surgery is usually performed before the cataracts harden, whereas the large-incision surgery is performed after the cataracts harden. Since the government doctors used the large-incision method of extracting cataracts, they preferred to wait longer to operate than a doctor would using the newer, no-stitch method.

Dr. Corboy pointed out that the term "unnecessary" cataract surgery was even dropped by Medicare in 1991 and replaced by "premature." However, since everyone will eventually need cataract surgery, the best time to operate is when the patient wishes to have it. Hence, when the doctors testified that Dr. Rutgard performed "unnecessary" cataract surgery, it simply meant that they would have waited six months or so longer until the cataract hardened before performing the older, riskier operation.

> Those who have judged Dr. Rutgard do not have the same surgical skills, therefore, they would counsel patients to wait longer. As The Academy of Ophthalmology points out in their Cataract Surgery brochure, "There is *no right or wrong opinion*, and ophthalmologists may have differing recommendations." Why would the board favor the opinion of lesser surgeons who have such a clear conflict of interest?[22]

Judicial Bias against Dr. Rutgard

Judicial bias in Dr. Rutgard's trial was so egregious that it is impossible to reconcile it with the American system of justice. Dr. Rutgard's rights were denied in two ways: incompetent defense counsel and a conviction based upon false evidence.

Even before Jeff Rutgard's criminal trial in 1995, he was denied due process of the law. Under the terms of the Sixth Amendment to the U.S. Constitution, any person who is accused of a crime has the right to "effective" legal counsel. The Fourteenth Amendment (due process clause) extends this right to state crimes. Dr. Rutgard's right to effective defense counsel was flagrantly violated by the Administrative Law Judge of the MBC and by the United States District Court of Southern California.

Jeff Rutgard hired attorney Richard Turner to represent him at the Administrative Law Hearing of the MBC. With four to six weeks to go in the hearing, Turner suffered a severe fracture of his leg requiring hospitalization and extensive surgery. He requested a postponement of the hearing because of his medical condition.

Turner told the judge, who was appointed by the prosecuting district attorney, that Rutgard's case involved thousands of documents, hundreds of witnesses, and required working 18 hours a day, 6 days a week. He said that every day he reviewed a 6- to 10-inch thick binder full of new materials, including complicated questions of medicine and medical techniques for the next day's hearings.

Turner informed the judge that if he were to continue in the case, it would jeopardize his health and Dr. Rutgard's defense. Despite his request and corroborating medical documentation, the Administrative Law Judge, Joyce Wharton, rejected Turner's request on the specious grounds that his injuries would not prevent him from attending the hearings.

Despite the judge's ruling, Turner withdrew from the case in February 1994. Rutgard was thus suddenly placed in the position of trying to get a competent replacement for his defense. Jeff Rutgard was turned down by numerous lawyers on the grounds that it would be impossible to step into the hearing at such a late date. They also said that it would take 10 to 12 months to prepare for his criminal trial. The upshot of this was that the perjured testimony of Rutgard's former employees was never questioned at the MBC hearing.

The tragic comedy of errors continued when Dr. Rutgard finally hired famed Texas criminal defense attorney, Richard "Racehorse" Haynes. Despite lacking expertise in medical fraud cases, Haynes agreed to step into the case at the end of the MBC administrative hearing. He also agreed to represent Rutgard at his trial for a fee of more than $600,000. Haynes' assistant received $200,000.

Jeff Rutgard told Haynes that his ex-employees and competitor doctors gave the MBC false testimony resulting in the suspension of his medical license. Haynes advised Dr. Rutgard to sue the ex-employees and the doctors in federal court to intimidate them into withdrawing their perjured testimony. On Haynes's advice, Dr. Rutgard sued his ex-employees and competing doctors in October 1992 on the grounds that they violated federal antitrust laws by trying to put Dr. Rutgard out of business. This backfired when the court threw the case out, asserting that it was meritless and frivolous since Rutgard's ex-employees were not competitors. The former employees, George Butera, Shirley Duncan, Mary Ellen Anderson, Kathy Diadezzio, and Jean Havel, then countersued Rutgard and Haynes under California law for malicious prosecution.

Since Haynes had not even taken depositions from the ex-employees or familiarized himself with the case, Rutgard was forced to settle with the employees by paying them huge damages. Haynes's insurer paid them $416,000, and Jeff Rutgard and his insurance company paid them $1.7 million to settle the lawsuit. The disgruntled employees each received $450,000 in damages. That was only the beginning of Dr. Rutgard's legal nightmare.

Just two weeks before Jeff Rutgard's criminal trial in October 1994, his attorneys admitted to the judge that they were not prepared for the trial. Haynes appealed to Federal District Judge, Gordon Thompson, to be relieved of his duty as Dr. Rutgard's lead counsel on the grounds that he could not render effective assistance to Dr. Rutgard.

Haynes pointed out that his assistant counsel, Juanita Brooks, was also not prepared to go to trial. Indeed, Ms. Brooks's later said that "two unprepared lawyers is better than one unprepared lawyer, which would have been me."[23] The judge denied Haynes and Brook's request and ordered them to proceed with the case. Nevertheless, Haynes withdrew from the case at the insistence of Dr. Rutgard in December 1994, and Brooks was forced to take over as the lead counsel.

The results of being unprepared for the case were predictable. Haynes and Brooks conducted lengthy, unfocused, and repetitive cross-examination of witnesses. Judge Thompson became so impatient that he openly ridiculed them in front of the jury.

For example, during the government's questioning of one of Dr. Rutgard's nurses regarding whether she entered patients' temperatures on the charts, the following exchange occurred between the judge and Haynes:[24]

> Mr. Haynes: Objection, if the Court please. The inclusion in the question fictitious is not the word of the witness, it's the word of the lawyer . . .
> The Court: Boy, you're a fine one to object to that. Objection is overruled.

When Haynes tried to ask a patient a question about injections that the government alleged did not occur, the judge said to Haynes, "Enough of the nonsense. Get on with the trial."[25] Judge Thompson also made repeated comments to the effect that if defense counsel did not like his rulings, then they could appeal it to the Ninth Circuit Court of Appeals.

The message to the jury was clear: Dr. Rutgard should be convicted. Judge Thompson also cut off Haynes's attempt to expose the false testimony of the disgruntled employees and limited the number of defense witnesses to 18 despite thousands of patients who were prepared to testify on behalf of Jeff Rutgard.

Furthermore, the judge ruled that the defense could not cross-examine the ex-employees about their malicious prosecution case that was pending at the time against Dr. Rutgard. Judge Thompson ruled that if Haynes brought this out in the court, the government could reveal to the jury that Dr. Rutgard's medical license had been revoked by the MBC. Since this would be highly prejudicial, Haynes did not cross-examine the former employees about their false testimony.

The Government's Case: Character Assassination

The prosecution's case was predicated upon destroying Dr. Rutgard's character. Neither the government nor Dr. Rutgard's defense presented evidence that he had violated any law or Medicare rule. Instead, the prosecution used the distorted anecdotes of his ex-employees and factual misrepresentation to make the preposterous claim that Rutgard's practice was so "permeated with fraud" that everything he did as a physician was criminal.

The government characterized Jeff Rutgard as a greedy, uncaring doctor whose primary motivation was self-enrichment at the public's expense. They told the jury that Dr. Rutgard instructed his staff to tell patients that "the Lord guides his work and skills." They said that the American College of Eye Surgeons had rebuked Dr. Rutgard for stating on his resume that he was a fellow rather than a member of the college. They said he gave patients copies of a book that showed him as a coauthor with Dr. Hoopes when, in fact, Rutgard paid to have his name added as the author. Prosecutors said that he gave his staff "quantifiable goals" to increase the number of operations he performed and that bonuses were given to the staff if they met these goals. The government said that Dr. Rutgard had sent $6.2 million (his entire family savings during 10 years of practice) out of the country as if he were a drug dealer engaged in money laundering.

The prosecution's distortion of fact and half truths were flagrant. For example, eye doctors, including the ones who testified against Dr. Rutgard, commonly provide free eye screenings at senior citizen centers. High-volume eye doctors also commonly give their employees bonuses for increased patient referrals. Dr. Hoopes, the coauthor of the ophthalmology book, asked Jeff Rutgard to read the book and supplement it with comments, and decided to add his name to the authorship of the book.

Given the prejudicial treatment that Dr. Rutgard received in the trial, it is not surprising that the jury convicted him on 130 counts of mail fraud, false claims, false statements, and money laundering. However, in a declaration by Fred Chavez, a juror in the trial, the biased nature of the government's strategy is evident. Chavez made the following statement:

> It is my feeling that the doctor did not have a chance with this jury. I felt that some of the witnesses against Dr. Rutgard lied under oath, and I didn't see anyone charged with perjury. I think that the jurors who were close to the doctor's age felt that he was making too much money. I changed my vote to "guilty" because of my concern over the cost of a retrial.[26]

A Draconian Sentence

Jeff Rutgard was convicted of fraudulently billing the government in the amount of $65,000. The prosecution got a conviction of Dr. Rutgard based upon billing Medicare for only 16 patients out of 22,000. This represents fewer than 0.1 percent of Jeff Rutgard's patients. Indeed, the judge observed near the end of the case that "over a four-or five-year period, you know, it's almost, to be honest with you, a minuscule amount of patients that you put on whose Medicare payments were fraudulent."[27] Nevertheless, the court gave Dr. Rutgard the most severe punishment possible. Based upon the OIG's extrapolation formula, Rutgard was found guilty of defrauding the government of $16 million, the entire amount paid to him by Medicare from the end of 1988 to April 1992. Under federal sentencing guidelines, prison sentences are based upon the dollar amount of the fraud, plus what are called "enhancements" or additional punishment. Each enhancement ranges between 3 and 12 months of prison time. Dr. Rutgard was given an additional 15 enhancements. He was given these enhancements because he was a doctor and was said to be guilty of an "abuse of trust" by victimizing Medicare and patients. Unlike street or violent criminals, he was given extra prison time precisely because he was a physician.

Jeff Rutgard received an 11 1/4-year prison sentence and ordered to pay restitution in the amount of $12 million. Despite the fact that his family was in California, he was sent as far away from them as possible to Fort Dix federal prison in New Jersey. His wife was forced to sell their home and move their five children to her parents' home in Iowa. Almost five years later, Dr. Rutgard successfully appealed his conviction and was released from prison. Nevertheless, as a convicted felon, he was stripped of his license to practice medicine and none of his family savings was returned to him. The government thus destroyed the career of a brilliant physician and has denied him the means to support his family.

A Political Scapegoat

The combination of being a high-volume eye surgeon and the federal and state prosecutorial traps made Jeff Rutgard an ideal political scapegoat. He was singled-out for prosecution as an example to all eye doctors. While other doctors in La Jolla were charged with defrauding Medicare they were not criminally prosecuted, however. For example, in 1990, Dr. Raymond Chan of La Jolla was charged with defrauding Medicare and ordered to pay a fine of $250,000. Unlike Dr. Rutgard, he did not lose his medical license and was allowed to continue in practice.

Indeed, only months before Dr. Rutgard was charged, San Diego prosecutors imposed a civil fine on the National Health Laboratories of La Jolla for defrauding Medicare by $250 million. This was the largest laboratory medical testing and pathology company in the country. Not only was the company allowed to stay in business but it was allowed to pay a civil fine over 10 years and the president of the company was only given a six-month sentence in the nicest prison camp in the country. By contrast, the same prosecutors told Dr. Rutgard that they would not accept a civil fine in his case and that he was going to prison for many years.

The outcome of Rutgard's case has had a chilling effect on all eye doctors in the country. The case has become a *cause celebre* for fraud investigators and prosecutors. Indeed, the OIG holds seminars featuring the Rutgard case.

The lesson is that to get a criminal conviction against a doctor all that is needed is collaborators in a doctor's office to turn them in for fraud and competing doctors to confirm that they have performed "unnecessary surgery." In other words, the government does not have to prove that a physician violated any law to obtain a criminal conviction. Self-serving hearsay evidence is sufficient to convict doctors of a criminal offense, seize their assets, and send them to prison.

TERRORIZING DOCTORS: GEORGE O. KRIZEK, M.D.

Dr. George Krizek was a dedicated 61-year-old psychiatrist working in Washington, DC, when he and his wife, Blanka, became the targets of a 12-year-long governmental investigation and prosecution for alleged fraud. The government claimed that they were guilty of fraudulently up-coding bills sent to Medicare and Medicaid for reimbursement in the amount of $245,392. Allegedly, the fraud was for "unnecessary medical treatment" in 8,002 individual claims. When the government multiplied each of the claims by a fine of $10,000, they came up with a colossal fine of $81 million.

Dr. Krizek's Devotion to Medicine

George Krizek worked tirelessly for 21 years in a major inner city hospital, the Washington Hospital Center (WHC), and had a small practice in his home. He worked seven days a week taking care of the poorest, sickest, and elderly patients. About 75 percent of his patients were Medicare or Medicaid, most of whom were sent to him by the emergency room of the hospital. These patients were seriously ill with multiple complications and had to be monitored almost daily. The Krizeks bought a dilapidated 100-year-old house within walking distance of the hospital so that he could be near his patients.

About 30 percent of Dr. Krizek's patients were charity cases for which he received no pay. From 1988 to 1992, the period of the indictment, George Krizek estimated he gave between 6,000 and 8,000 hours of free care to indigent patients. In addition to the psychiatric conditions of his patients, many had life-threatening conditions such as brain hemorrhage, AIDS, diabetes, and drug addiction. Most psychiatrists would not treat these patients. Indeed, fewer than 30 percent of all psychiatrists see patients like these. The psychiatrist who testified for the government against Dr. Kriezk at his trial, Dr. Harvey Resnik, did not even accept Medicare and Medicaid patients.

George Krizek frequently worked nights, weekends, and holidays at the hospital covering for other psychiatrists who were on vacation or were away for the weekend. He felt that he had an obligation to his newly adopted country to serve the poorest and sickest people in society when others would not. Dr. Krizek described the crisis in psychiatry in the United States. He said that hundreds of thousands of psychiatric beds have been abolished. Psychiatric hospitals have been closed and people who need care have been sent out on the streets. They do not get treatment, medication, food, and many are in the drug business and some have AIDS.

Despite working 70 or 80 hours a week, Dr. Krizek had an average gross income of about $100,000 per year. After office expenses and malpractice insurance, it left him with a net income of about $70,000. His wife Blanka, who managed the paperwork in his home office, received no pay at all for her work. She did not even contribute to her social security retirement account.

As a result of the government's investigation and prosecution of Dr. Krizek, his medical practice, economic livelihood, family security, and even his physical health was destroyed. George Krizek was forced to close his practice and all of his family assets, including his home, were frozen. Dr. Krizek lost his ability to earn a living and soon after the trial, he was diagnosed with cancer. He and his wife did not even have money enough to pay for their own medical treatment.

Because of his trial, Krizek was unable to see his 87-year-old mother in the Czech Republic before she died. Ironically, the collapse of Communism in 1992 made it possible for George Krizek to visit his mother, a widow of a resistance fighter, for the first time since he fled the country in 1966. However, she died before he had an opportunity to see her. She passed away with the knowledge that her son was being prosecuted by the very country in which he sought political freedom.

Escape from Communist Oppression

Dr. Krizek fled his native Czechoslovakia in 1966, after being ordered to join the Communist party and carry out politically motivated psychiatric investigations of enemies of the state. He managed to get his wife and child out of the country in 1967 and after the Soviet Union and Warsaw Pact forces invaded Czechoslovakia in 1968, he fulfilled his lifelong dream of starting a new life of freedom in America. Dr. Krizek became a naturalized U.S. citizen in 1974.

When Dr. Krizek arrived in the United States, he had a medical degree from Charles University School of Medicine in Prague. He also qualified to practice medicine at the Vienna Medical School in Austria and served as the chief psychiatrist at the prestigious Charles University Psychiatric Outpatient Clinic.

Krizek completed a two-year psychiatric residency in the United States at Beth Israel Medical Center in New York City specializing in substance abuse disorders. He started working in Washington, DC, at the Washington Hospital Center in 1972, and was certified by the American Board of Psychiatry and Neurology in 1977.

Background of the Prosecution

Dr. Krizek's prosecution occurred shortly after Congress amended the False Claims Act in 1986. The original act was adopted in 1863, by Abraham Lincoln, during the civil war. The act enabled "whistleblowers," called "relators" or *qui tam* plaintiffs (citizen suits), to collect up to 35 percent of fraudulent monies recovered by the government.

The act remained virtually unchanged for 123 years until President Reagan came to power in the 1980s. The Reagan administration increased military spending and at the same time called for reducing the role of government. This focused media attention upon combating government fraud.

To that end, Congress strengthened the False Claims Act in 1986, and made it the government's principal weapon against fraud. The act increased penalties for fraud from $2,000 for each false claim to between $5,000 and $10,000 for each claim plus three times the amount of the fraud.

The act eliminated the need to prove specific intent to commit defraud. "Deliberate ignorance" or "reckless disregard" of the truth was now sufficient to prove fraud.

The act gave the government greater flexibility in prosecuting fraud. They could now bring criminal or civil charges against an accused or use an internal administrative law proceeding. In other words, if the government lost a criminal case, it could sue in a civil court, or it could submit the case to their own administrative law judge. This placed the accused in danger of "triple jeopardy." In effect, it meant that the government was almost certain to win fraud cases.

Soon after the amendment, health became the principal target of the government's false-claims prosecutions. For example, from 1988 to 1992, health care cases accounted for 15 percent of all new *qui tam* cases. By 1998, 61 percent of all new cases involved allegations of health care fraud.[28]

The Government Targets Dr. Krizek

The investigation of the Krizeks began soon after the passage of the amended False Claims Act. George Krizek was the first psychiatrist in the Washington, DC, area to be investigated for submitting false claims. The OIG wanted a high-profile case to inaugurate its newly acquired prosecutorial powers. George Krizek presented just such an opportunity for testing the act.

The OIG ordered an investigation of Dr. Krizek as early as 1987. The OIG headquarters office of investigations asked the regional OIG audit office in Washington, DC, for a billing profile of Dr. Krizek. This is contrary to the standard investigative procedure.

Fraud cases are supposed to be discovered first by the audit department. Billing errors are next supposed to be brought to the attention of the physician concerned. Only if a billing discrepancy cannot be reconciled with the physician, is it to be turned over to the OIG's office for investigation.

In Dr. Krizek's case, this procedure was ignored entirely. The OIG's office of investigation initiated the investigation instead of the audit department and it was never brought to Dr. Krizek's attention. The prosecution tried to mislead the court by saying that the OIG's audit department had first uncovered a high computer billing profile for Dr. Krizek when it conducted a study of psychiatrist's use of a single CPT code—90844 (comprehensive individual psychotherapy).[29] During the trial, however, the judge insisted upon seeing the evidence. After threatening to dismiss the case, the OIG finally produced a computer print-out of George's Krizek's billing record.

The judge discovered that two-thirds of the 600 Washington-area (Pennsylvania, New Jersey, Delaware and the District of Columbia, and parts of Maryland and Virginia) psychiatrists used the 90844 code more often than did Dr. Krizek for the same kind of treatment. Some psychiatrists received up to five times more money from Medicare and Medicaid than did Dr. Krizek. The judge wanted to know why the government had singled him out for prosecution. The prosecutor lamely responded that Krizek was being sued because his billing profile was high.

The Investigation Begins

The Krizeks's ordeal began on December 12, 1989, when Mrs. Krizek received an anonymous phone call asking if she would be home that evening "to receive a Christmas delivery." Shortly after the call, three special agents of the OIG arrived unannounced at their home. Two of the agents were former FBI agents in undercover counterintelligence surveillance.[30] Blanka Krizek was expecting a large poinsettia plant that a grateful patient and friend sent the Krizeks every Christmas. Instead of the poinsettia plant, three large investigators, two men and a woman, appeared on her doorstep. For several hours, they accused Blanka and George Krizek of double-billing, billing for nondelivered services, and "enriching themselves." The agents bullied, intimidated, and made fun of her accent.

Mrs. Krizek was scared to death. The agents presented her with a list of what they described as "non-existent" patients and demanded the files. Terrified and shaking, she found the files and handed them over. Blanka Krizek later described the experience as the most "unpleasant experience in (her) quarter of a century (in America)."

The presiding judge at the trial, Stanley Sporkin, admonished the investigators for running a "gumshoe operation." He castigated them for not identifying themselves when they called on the Krizeks and not producing a subpoena when they arrived.

> This is not the way a legitimate agency of the US Government conducts an investigation, say we got a delivery to make and the delivery happens to be a Xerox machine to take copies of records. You never gave them the subpoena that you said you had to give them.[31]

The agents also went to the Washington Hospital Center and questioned Dr. Krizek's associates and patients about his "fraudulent" billing and "medically unnecessary" services. However, they could not find a single doctor, nurse, or patient to testify against Dr. Krizek. Indeed, over 50 professional colleagues at the WHC were unwilling to offer any testimony against him. In fact, several testified at the trial in his defense.

Despite having no documentation of fraudulent behavior and no witnesses, the government nevertheless decided to prosecute the Krizeks. The government did not communicate with them from 1989 to 1992. Neither Medicare, nor Medicaid, nor the insurance company, Pennsylvania Blue Shield, which processed the claims, notified Dr. Krizek of any incorrect billing.

In December 1992, the U.S. Attorney's Office for the District of Columbia sent the Krizeks a threatening letter out of the blue demanding $400,000 for "fraudulent billing" or face prosecution. The Krizeks rejected the government's demand. They not only had not committed fraud, but they had nowhere near that amount of money.

The government responded by calling a hastily organized press conference on January 11, 1993. Jay Stevens, the U.S. Attorney for Washington, DC, told the media that the government was filing a lawsuit against Dr. Krizek and his wife for submitting 8,002 fraudulent bills to Medicare and Medicaid, with potential fines of $81 million. Throughout the day and evening, television and radio stations ran stories dramatizing the Krizeks's fraud against the health care system that protected the elderly and poor. They described the Krizek's 100-year-old renovated home as a castle and showed shots of it on TV from a news helicopter hovering in the sky above.

The Case against the Krizeks

The OIG originally wanted to criminally prosecute the Krizeks; however, the U.S. Attorney's Office rejected that because they did not have enough evidence. Instead of dropping the case, however, the OIG decided to bring a civil lawsuit against the Krizeks.

George and Blanka Krizek were charged with two types of fraudulent misconduct. The first was that Dr. Krizek "up-coded" bills for 20 to 30 minutes of patient treatment (CPT 98043 for office and CPT 90862 for hospital visits). Instead of billing the government for 20 to 30 minute patient treatment, he charged for 45 to 50 minutes (CPT 90844). The government prosecutor referred to the 45 to 50 minute treatment as the "Cadillac" code and implied that Dr. Krizek was charging for a Cadillac but was only delivering a Hyundai.

Despite this claim, Dr. Krizek only received an average of $21 per Medicaid patient and $45 per Medicare patient. He received about $362.50 a year for each Medicare patient he saw in his office. If Dr. Krizek saw the patient once a month, that would mean he received $30.20 per visit, and if he saw them twice a month, he would be reimbursed $15.10 per visit. This contrasted with the government's expert witness in the trial, Dr. Harvey Reznik, who received $250 per patient visit up front.

The second allegation was that Dr. Krizek performed 8,002 unnecessary medical services from 1988 to 1992. Since it was not feasible to evaluate all of these cases, the court decided to consider seven of George Krizek's patients.

The Judge Questions the Charges

The government took the position that Dr. Krizek could not legally bill for a 45- to 50-minute code (CPT 90844) unless he spent his entire time with a patient. In other words, if Dr. Krizek spent 25 minutes in the presence of a patient and then spent an additional 20 minutes discussing the case with another doctor or nurse out of sight of the patient, he could not legally bill for the 45 minute code.

Judge Sporkin was skeptical of the government's case from the beginning. During the first day of the trial, for example, the judge made the following comment. He said that nowhere in the 45–50-minute code does it say the doctor has to be "face to face" with a patient in order to bill for the time spent with the patient.

The judge was outraged when he discovered that doctors who saw patients in the hospital could bill for only one code a day despite providing many services such as reviewing laboratory results, X-Rays, speaking with therapists, family members, prescribing medication. Sporkin said that if the government's case against Dr. Krizek was that he used the wrong billing code and if they held doctors to this standard, "We're going to have no doctors working in this country anymore."[32]

Judge Sporkin elaborated by saying that if the government gave him a test on the rules of criminal procedure, "I'd flunk because I don't know what Rule 142 says or Rule 144; you can't hold doctors to this kind of standard."[33] The judge was so infuriated that he accused the government of committing fraud against doctors. Sporkin said,

> You don't tell a doctor to put in two claims and then say, "But, we're only going to pay you for one." That's not only fraud; that's dishonesty. Our government is being fraud operators; we've got a serious problem in this country.[34]

Dr. Krizek provided a wide range of treatment for his patients and billed for a single 45- to 50-minute code even though he often spent more than an hour with them. For example, George Krizek often treated patients with Munchhausen syndrome. These are patients who seek medical treatment for imaginary ailments or diseases. One such patient came to the hospital claiming to have swallowed two razor blades. Doctors were going to operate when Dr. Krizek intervened and told the surgeons that the patient had made similar claims before and they were untrue.

The patient had previously claimed that he had stomach cancer, colon cancer, brain atrophy, deteriorated knees plus other diseases. He invented diseases and aliments and then searched for doctors who would treat them. Invariably, just before a doctor was ready to operate, the patient said that he did not have these aliments.

In addition to Munchhausen syndrome, the patient did have real diseases. He was an alcoholic, had an enlarged prostrate, had blood in his urine, kidney stones, lung cancer, and eye illnesses. Dr. Krizek had to deal with his Munch-hausen syndrome plus all of his other diseases and coordinate his treatment with other doctors and nurses. For this combined treatment, Krizek could bill for only one service. The logical billing code was CPT 90844 because it came the closest to the time he spent treating the patient.

Unjust Conviction: A False Analogy

Judge Sporkin dismissed most of the charges against the Krizeks. He found Dr. Krizek not guilty of providing "unnecessary medical treatment." He said that George Krizek was a competent and capable doctor who worked long hours on behalf of patients most of whom had "horribly severe psychiatric disorders and other serious medical conditions."[35]

Judge Sporkin found the Krizeks guilty of violating the False Claims Act, however. He said that attorneys bill for services rendered at 10-minute inter-vals and would not, as a rule, bill for more than nine hours a day. He found the Krizeks guilty of "gross negligence" for submitting bills to the government that exceed nine patient-treatment hours a day.

Such billing practices may well work in the legal profession. However, they certainly do not work in the practice of medicine. Most physicians regularly work 12 or more hours a day including weekends. Unlike the practice of law, medicine is not a nine-to-five job. Physicians routinely treat patients at night and on weekends.

As Dr. Krizek testified, he frequently worked 24-hour shifts in the hospital covering for doctors who were off duty. Judge Sporkin's ruling was not only unprecedented, but if doctors were ordered to follow it, the country's health care system would collapse.

Destruction of the Krizek Family

Blanka and George Krizek sought to appeal their conviction of violating the False Claims Act. They appealed the case to the District Court of Appeals. In October 2000, the Appeals Court rejected the Krizeks's case without hear-ing their legal arguments and the U.S. Supreme Court refused to hear the case.

The impact of the Krizeks's legal ordeal had taken a high toll on them. As a result of Judge Sporkin's ruling, Dr. Krizek was not allowed to submit bills for Medicare and Medicaid claims. Since most of his patients were Medicare and Medicaid it meant that he was unable to practice medicine. He became depressed and despondent over his conviction and in January 1996 developed cancer.

At the time that Dr. Krizek was diagnosed with cancer and operated on, his daughter met with the assistant U.S. Attorney. She told him about her father's illness and asked the government to remove the freeze on their assets so they could pay for medical treatment and support themselves. She was greeted by stony silence and escorted out of the building under armed guard.

The government refused to accept the $157,000 fine ordered by Judge Sporkin. The U.S. Attorney appealed the judge's decision claiming that Dr. Krizek should pay $5,745,000 in fines that are required under the False Claims Act.

The Krizeks appealed to Judge Sporkin for relief. The judge responded to the Krizeks's impassioned plea by asking what the government wanted. Sporkin said the case could be settled in 10 or 15 minutes. However, the government refused to say what they wanted from the Krizeks.

Privately, the assistant U.S. Attorney who prosecuted the case told the Krizeks that since the government offered to settle the case for $400,000 before the trial, that would be the starting point for negotiations after the trial that they won. He added that if the Krizeks did not have the money, the government would settle for less. In September 2002, Monika Krizek mortgaged her home and used her savings to settle the case by paying the government $315,000.

CHARLES T. SELL, D.D.S.: IMPRISONMENT WITHOUT TRIAL

Dr. Charles "Tom" Sell, D.D.S., was a 48-year-old dentist with a successful 17-year practice in Town and Country, an upscale suburb of St. Louis, Missouri, when he became a victim of the government's overzealous fraud investigation. Tom Sell graduated from the University of Missouri Dental School in 1976. He was married with two young children. His wife, Mary Sell, was the office manager who handled all the billing. The Sells were sent to prison without trial, Mary for $4^1/_2$ months and Tom for almost 8 years, including 20 months in solitary confinement. Due to legal expenses, he lost his practice, office, home, and savings.

In 1982, Tom Sell was treated for a "delusional disorder." He was given an antidepressant, Parozetine, returned to work and led a normal home and work life without incident until he was arrested by the FBI in 1997. Sell was also a major in the U.S. Army Reserve specializing in forensic dentistry and a member of the ultraconservative Missouri-based Council of Conservative Citizens (CCC). Dr. Sell advertised his dental services on a CCC Web site and on a radio program hosted by Gordon Baum, the executive officer of the CCC. The CCC has campaigned against forced busing of public school children in Saint Louis and affirmative action, among other issues.

The CCC has been accused of being racist, but its leaders insist that they are simply advocating white rights in the same way that the National Association for the Advancement of Colored People advocates the rights of blacks. Senator Trent Lott (R-Miss) received notoriety for his membership in the Mississippi chapter of the CCC.

Investigation and Arrest of Dr. Sell

In April 1997, the FBI simultaneously raided the Sells's home and office and seized patient records and documents. One month later, Dr. Sell was arrested for Medicaid fraud. At the time of Dr. Sell's arrest, he was treating Medicaid patients in his office. Tom Sell told the judge that the charges were a mistake. He said he treated Medicaid patients only one day a week and did not make money from it. He cared for impoverished patients largely out of charity.

Dr. Sell explained that if patients' front teeth were weak, Medicaid would only pay to pull them out. However, he refused to pull their teeth and bonded them instead with a filling and charged the government for the service. He also refused to collect a copayment from the patients, as required by Medicaid, because they could not afford it. When questioned about these practices, Dr. Sell simply said, "What's wrong with that?"[36]

In July 1997, a federal grand jury indicted Tom and Mary Sell on five counts of fraud for making false statements from 1989 to 1997 on bills submitted to the government for reimbursement. Dr. Sell vehemently denied any wrongdoing and insisted that the FBI had targeted him for prosecution because of public statements he had made about the deadly fire at the Branch Davidian compound in Waco, Texas, on April 19, 1993, that killed 80 people, including 22 children. Dr. Sell said he was at the site of the Waco compound on the day of the tragic fire.

Sell claims that the government deliberately fire-bombed the Davidian compound and was responsible for the deaths of dozens of innocents. Sell feared that the FBI wanted him dead in order to silence him. Army records show that he was, indeed, activated by the Army on April 19, 1993, and assigned to Fort Sam Houston in San Antonio, which is near the Davidian compound. However, they would not confirm that he was at the site of the compound.

Since Dr. Sell had a history of "delusional disorder" and advocated a conspiracy theory of the Waco fire, the judge ordered him to undergo psychological evaluation at the Springfield prison hospital to determine his competence to stand trial. Springfield had a notorious reputation that was uncovered by a "60 Minutes" report in 1991, alleging that the hospital's mistreatment of inmates caused "unnecessary death and disfigurement." Springfield is primarily a prison and only secondarily a hospital.

After he arrived at Springfield in 1997, Sell attended a mental competency course and took a 30-question true/false written test used in the prison Competency Restoration Group. The test was designed to determine whether he understood the charges against him, could assist in his defense, and therefore was competent to stand trial.

Dr. Richard L. DeMier, the clinical psychologist at Springfield prison, administered the test and wrote a letter to the court stating that Dr. Sell had passed the mental competency course, received a perfect score on the test, and was mentally fit to stand trial. Tom Sell was released on bond on August 1997, after spending three months in prison. He returned to Saint Louis to be with his family and resume working. He was required to wear an electronic ankle detection bracelet pending his trial, however.

In November 1997, the government increased Sell's indictment from 5 felony counts to 63 counts of insurance and Medicaid fraud. The increase in felony counts was undoubtedly designed to intensify the government's leverage over Tom Sell to accept a plea bargain.

Indeed, on December 1, 1997, the government offered the Sells a plea bargain to settle the case. The U.S. Attorney, Edward L. Dowd, Jr., offered to drop the charges if Tom Sell would plead guilty to one count of mail fraud and one count of Medicaid fraud and Mary sell would plead guilty to one count of making a false claim. They would also have to pay a civil fine.

Dr. Sell rejected the offer, insisting on his innocence, and demanded a trial to prove it. On January 30, 1998, the chief prosecutor in the case and assistant U.S. Attorney, Dorthy L. McMurtry, offered Tom Sell another plea bargain. She asked Dr. Sell's attorney, Barry Short, if Sell would plead guilty to "something" in return for favorable treatment of his wife, Mary.[37] Dr. Sell again rejected the offer and demanded a trial to prove his innocence.

Dr. Sell's Re-arrest on Hearsay Evidence

On January 23, 1998, Tom Sell was re-arrested when he appeared for a scheduled meeting with his probation officer at the U.S. courthouse in Saint Louis. He was jailed on the grounds that he violated the conditions of his pretrial release. The government claimed that Dr. Sell broke his agreement to "avoid all contact with persons who are alleged victims or potential witnesses" in his fraud case.

The charge was based on an unsubstantiated complaint by Jane Ann Alderman, Dr. Sell's former dental assistant and his principal accuser in the fraud case. Alderman was originally placed in Dr. Sell's office by FBI agent Anthony Box in order to obtain information to bring fraud charges against the Sells.

The FBI persuaded Alderman to be a whistleblower in Dr. Sell's office as a condition for going easy on her for lying at a workers' compensation hearing and giving misleading information to the Drug Enforcement Agency. She was ideal for the task since she previously worked in medical offices and reportedly was a whistleblower against another doctor.

Alderman claimed that after Dr. Sell was released on bond, he visited her office building and stood about 60 feet outside of her office "waving and shaking his finger at me shaped like a gun; he was also smiling."[38] Alderman stated that she "freaked-out" and ran to call FBI Agent Box to report that Dr. Sell had threatened her life. She later gave agent Box a one-page handwritten note accusing Dr. Sell of threatening her life. This letter became exhibit A in Tom Sell's court hearing.

The FBI did not investigate Alderman's complaint, and the defense did not have an opportunity to question her at the hearing. The judge simply accepted her hearsay evidence, despite the prosecution's admission that Dr. Sell had said nothing to Alderman, did not approach her, and did not enter the office where she worked. The improbable nature of Jane Alderman's accusation raises serious questions as to whether the incident ever actually occurred.

For example, Jane Alderman claimed that she was sitting at the front desk at Premier Dental Group on the second floor of a three-story building and saw Dr. Sell "no more than 60 feet away looking at me through the glass window." When defense attorney Barry Short asked FBI Agent Box where Dr. Sell would have been if he were 60 feet away from Alderman, Agent Box answered that he did not know.

Anthony Box also admitted that Dr. Sell was ordered by the court to visit his therapist, Dr. Jay Englehart, whose office was located in the same building and on the same floor as the Premier Dental Group office. On the day of the alleged threat, Tom Sell made his fourth visit to Dr. Englehart's office. The elevator is less than 20 feet away from the Premier Dental Group office, and Dr. Englehart's office is between 20 and 30 feet, or three doors, from the Premier Dental office. Agent Box could not explain Sell's estimated 60-foot distance from Alderman, nor did he know whether it was even possible for Jane Alderman to see down the corridor from the front desk of Premier Dental Group.

Furthermore, Tom Sell was driven to the office building by his wife, Mary Sell, and accompanied by one of their sons. Mary Sell testified that she dropped off her husband at the office building at 2:30 P.M., saw him in the lobby of the building before his appointment with Dr. Englehart, and promptly picked him up after his appointment at 3:00 P.M.

Alderman claims that Dr. Sell threatened her at 3:30 P.M. that afternoon. Incredulously, Alderman also claimed that three days before the alleged incident, she thought that Tom and Mary Sell followed her to work. However, she conceded in her statement that "this might be just my imagination."

Politically Incorrect Behavior and Judicial Bias

Tom Sell was outraged by his arrest at the courthouse on January 23, 1998, and demanded to see his attorney, who was out of town at the time. Sell was angry, highly emotional, and used the "N word" several times making reference to FBI Agent Anthony Box and assistant U.S. Attorney, Dorothy McMurtry, the chief prosecutor of his fraud case.

Box and McMurtry were African-Americans and were in the courthouse at the time of Dr. Sell's arrest and heard his outburst. The judge, Mary Ann L. Medler, also overheard Sell's flare-up and made the following statement about it at his court hearing three days later on January 26, 1998:

> I could hear (*Dr. Sell*) screaming, shouting, frequently using the (N) word. It was most offensive to me. I proceeded to Sell's holding cell. I stood outside of his cell, but before I could begin, Dr. Sell began screaming, shouting raging, directing personal insults at me, and shouting for his attorney. I tried to advise him of his rights, but he reared forward and spat directly into my face.[39]

At the beginning of Tom Sell's hearing, Barry Short, his attorney, asked the judge to recuse herself. Short argued that in light of the spitting incident and Sell's use of obscenities, the judge's impartiality could be questioned. Short cited U.S.C. S455 that reads:

(a) Any justice, judge, or magistrate of the United States should disqualify himself in any proceeding in which his impartiality might reasonably be questioned.
(b) He shall also disqualify himself in the following circumstances: (1) Where he has a personal bias or prejudice concerning a party.

Short also discussed Congress's 1974 "objective" standard for determining a judge's impartiality. The standard

asks what a reasonable person knowing all of the relevant facts would think about the impartiality or the judge *even where the question is close*, the judge whose impartiality might reasonably be questioned must recuse himself from the trial.[40]

Despite the U.S. legal code and the clear intention of Congress, Judge Medler refused to recuse herself and presided over Dr. Sell's hearing.

At the conclusion of the hearing, the judge revoked Dr. Sell's bond and ordered him jailed on the grounds that his testimony was "self-serving" and not credible. She also said that he posed a danger to himself and the safety of the community.[41] The judge arrived at this conclusion despite the fact that Sell's therapist, Dr. Englehart, never reported that Dr. Sell was a danger to anyone. In fact, Englehart said that Tom Sell was "verbalizing anger and some delusion stories but he was fine."[42] It is noteworthy that delusional disorder is a new and rare diagnosis and is not well understood by psychiatrists. Indeed, it was first diagnosed as a mental illness in 1987.

One must ask whether the judge would have described Tom Sell as dangerous, requiring incarceration, if were not for the spitting and obscenity incident. The significance of the judge's remark cannot be exaggerated. In all subsequent legal proceedings, this was described as an assault against a federal judge. Indeed, during a U.S. Supreme Court hearing of the Sell case in April 2003, Associate Justice Ruth Bader Ginsberg commented that Dr. Sell sounds dangerous. Thus, Judge Medler's ruling provided a government rationale for keeping Dr. Sell in jail for almost 8 years without a trial.

Indictment for Murder Conspiracy

On April 23, 1998, three months after Dr. Sell was rearrested, the government indicted him and his wife for conspiracy to murder Jane Alderman and FBI Agent Anthony Box. The government entered a six-count murder conspiracy indictment against the Sells. However, the evidence for the charges were just a flimsy as the alleged finger-pointing threat to Alderman.

The government's evidence for the murder conspiracy is a six-hour FBI audio tape recorded by two of Dr. Sell's acquaintances purporting to show that Tom and Mary Sell conspired to kill FBI agent Box and Jane Alderman. The FBI secretly recorded conversations between Tom and Mary Sell and the children of a friend and long-tern patient, Jonathan and Rebecca Gamble—who were brother and sister.

The government claimed that the tapes were evidence of murder conspiracy. Exactly what the tapes reveal, however, is subject to interpretation. The Sells claim that the tapes only show that they were trying to get information on Jane Alderman and the FBI agent that would exonerate Dr. Sell in the fraud case. The government claims, on the other hand, that a recorded comment by Dr. Sell to Jonathan Gamble, "If you're going to do it. Go for the big guy, man" is evidence of murder conspiracy. Tom and Mary Sell insist that this comment was made to encourage the Gambles to gather information about a conspiracy between FBI agent and Alderman in the Sells's Medicaid fraud case. Given Dr. Sell's delusional disorder, their explanation is quite plausible.

Moreover, the credibility of the Gambles is in serious doubt. For example, in the 1990s, Rebecca Gamble filed a complaint that she had been harassed for years by a Saint Louis union leader. The union leader was jailed based upon her testimony. Gamble publicly repeated her allegations against the union boss on Geraldo Rivera's national TV show. However, in 1997, a Jefferson County judge reversed the conviction of the union leader and ordered Gamble to pay him $513,000 for malicious prosecution.

Even more doubtful is the supposed incentive for the murder conspiracy. The prosecution claims that in February 1998, one month after Dr. Sell was rearrested, Mary Sell gave the Gambles $235 as a "down payment" for a hitman to carry out a double homicide. It strains credibility to believe that such a trivial amount of money would be sufficient to hire an assassin. More likely is Mary Sell's claim that she gave the Gambles money to cover the costs of gathering and photocopying evidence of a conspiracy by Alderman and the FBI in the Sells's Medicaid case.

The Case for Sell's Violence and Incompetence

The medical staff at Springfield prison manufactured a case to fit Judge Medler's verdict. Judge Medler ruled that Dr. Sell was a danger to himself and the community and, therefore, should be jailed. In order to justify this verdict, the staff had to reverse their 1997 assessment that Dr. Sell was competent to stand trial and was not dangerous. Dr. Richard L. MeMier was the staff clinical psychologist, and Dr. James K. Wolfson was the staff psychiatrist at Springfield. They worked together, however. Dr. Wolfson spent less than six hours with Dr. Sell and he entered only one sentence in Tom Sell's patient file.

Between February and March of 1999, Dr. MeMier and an intern, Paul Zahn, did another assessment of Dr. Sell. They prepared a report based upon this evaluation of Tom Sell's mental state on April 7, 1999, for the U.S. District

Court for the Eastern District of Missouri, which was held the following week. In the report, DeMier contradicted his earlier 1997 report and concluded that Tom Sell suffered from a "prosecutorial type" of delusional disorder and, therefore, was incompetent to stand trial. He also said that Dr. Sell was dangerous and should be medicated.

The absurdity of Dr. DeMier's position was his testimony at an involuntary medication hearing before the U.S. Eastern District court on September 29, 1999. He said that no one was certain who ordered Dr. Sell into isolation or why he was there.[43] Under questioning, however, he admitted that he was responsible for placing Dr. Sell in solitary confinement. Dr. DeMier did this despite acknowledging that Dr. Sell had not exhibited any assaultive behavior or threatened anyone.

Dr. DeMier insisted that Tom Sell was dangerous and must be placed in solitary until he took antipsychotic medication to restore his competence to stand trial. DeMier was adamant that Dr. Sell be medicated despite the fact that he was not qualified to prescribe the medication and he had treated only two inmates before with antipsychotic drugs. Indeed, Dr. DeMier acknowledged that only one of the inmates was restored to competency.

Despite conflicting medical testimony. Dr. DeMier and Dr. James K. Wolfson, the prison's consulting psychiatrist, contended that Tom Sell could become competent if he took a powerful, and potentially dangerous, antipsychotic drug.

Dr. Sell vehemently objected to his forced drugging with powerful mind-altering drugs. The defense's psychiatrist, Dr. C. Robert Cloninger, a professor and chair of the Department of Psychiatry at Washington University, disagreed with both DeMier and Wolfson's recommendation that Dr. Sell be forcibly drugged. Dr. Cloninger testified that the administration of antipsychotic drugs such as Olanzapine could prove fatal to Dr. Sell.

Furthermore, these drugs could produce permanent symptoms, such as shaking comparable to Parkinson's disease. Dr. Sell had, in fact, taken Haldol, an antipsychotic drug briefly in 1982, and it produced muscle spasms. Dr. Cloninger also explained that antidepressants and psychotherapy were the best treatment for delusional disorder, not antipsychotic drugs. Furthermore, he felt that the isolation of Dr. Sell would be the worst possible treatment.

Dr. Wolfson disputed Dr. Cloninger's testimony and insisted that the administration of antipsychotic drugs was the only treatment that could restore Dr. Sell's competence to stand trial. DeMier took the position that Tom Sell had to be kept in isolation until he agreed to take the antipsychotic drugs. The government offered to drop nearly 60 counts of Medicaid and mail fraud and money laundering against him in exchange for a guilty plea of two counts. Not long after Sell refused the offer, the government began trying to medicate Sell.[44] Based upon DeMier's report, the U.S. District Court ruled that Dr. Sell was dangerous and ordered him to take the antipsychotic medication. DeMier's contention that Dr. Sell was dangerous was based upon two flimsy complaints. The first is that Tom Sell warned Dr. DeMier that he should be prepared to testify in Congress about Dr. Sell's case.[45] The second is a written complaint by Michelle Goldenberg, a nurse who treated Dr. Sell at Springfield. She was selected by Dr. Sell as his staff representative at his institutional involuntary medication hearing. She was someone in whom Tom Sell had trust.

In July 1999, Goldenberg wrote a complaint about Dr. Sell's behavior, stating that he had asked her for an aspirin and then tried to talk to her. She told Sell that she had no time to talk to him, and he responded that she "never had time for him anymore." Goldenberg ordered Dr. Sell to leave the nursing station, and he called her by her first name. The report read as follows:

> Inmate came to nurse's station for aspirin, he wanted to continue talking with this writer (*Michele Goldenberg*), and I told him I didn't have time. He stated, "You never have time for me anymore; I'm not special anymore." He proceeded to tell this writer, "You just don't realize what you mean to me." Inmate was given a direct order to leave, that his behavior was out of line. He then stated, "I can't help myself." He has approached this writer in the past and stated, "Hello, Michelle." He has been reprimanded before for his inappropriate behavior towards this writer.[46]

In a twist of irony, Dr. DeMier had to contradict himself once more in order to justify the court's ruling that Dr. Sell was dangerous. In July 1999, he declared that Tom Sell was competent to participate in a prison disciplinary hearing. This occurred in response to Goldenberg's complaint. The prison warden, Bill Hedrick, made the following statement regarding Dr. Sell's competency to appear before a prison disciplinary hearing:

> A psychologist (*Dr. DeMier*) evaluated your condition (*Dr. Sell*), and determined that you are legally responsible for your behavior, and that you are competent to participate in disciplinary proceeding before the Unit Disciplinary committee.[47]

Four days after the disciplinary hearing, Tom Sell was placed in "lock down" or solitary confinement, where he remained for almost two years.

The Brutality of Confinement in 10E

Confinment in the 10E living unit of Springfield is the most brutal and violent in the entire prison. Inmates are kept in a 6 by 10-foot cell with only a bunk and a toilet. They remain there 23 hours a day and are allowed to exercise only 1 hour a day by themselves under strict observation. They are fed in their cells. Trays of food are pushed through a slot in a steel door. Prisoners are not allowed to have glasses with metal frames, and the prison does not provide glasses with plastic frames. Inmates cannot control the lights in their cells. They are permitted to have the use of a pencil to write, but they have to request it, and it is only brought around once a day. Before the cell door is opened, inmates must turn their backs to the door, put their hands behind their backs, and place them through the slot in the cell door for handcuffing. They are allowed to take a shower every other day.

One incident will illustrate the cruel treatment received by Dr. Sell while in solitary confinement. The events described below were witnessed by three Bureau of Prisons officials and five inmates. The Bureau of Prisons officials were nurse Michele Goldenberg, officer Laura Lee Bell, and officer Clay. The inmates were Edward Fluher, Scott Hatfield, Tyrone Anderson, Payne, and Alsell. There was also a videotape recording of the events.

On November 9, 1999, after four months in solitary and while alone in his cell, Tom Sell threw an empty plastic food tray against the wall. Under the pretext that Dr. Sell intended to use the pieces of the tray as a weapon, a squad of six guards assembled outside his cell.

Seeing the guards, Tom Sell placed his hands behind his back and stuck them through a slot in the door to be handcuffed. After he was handcuffed and without resisting, the guards burst through the door, wrestled him to the ground and took him to a cell on a lower floor of the prison. He was injected with a drug, against court order, and had his clothes removed except for his undershorts. Dr. Sell was handcuffed to a metal "black box" wrapped around his waist by chains that were connected to ankle shackles and laid on a concrete slab. For the next 19 1/2 hours, Tom Sell remained locked in that position on the slab. The cuff and ankle shackles were so tight that they cut through his skin and caused severe swelling. As a result of the pain, the effects of the drug, and lack of good blood circulation, Tom Sell passed in and out of consciousness.

Dr. Sell overheard nurse Goldenberg say that if his restrains were not loosened, he would not survive another 24 hours. He also heard Dr. DeMier screaming the question, "Will you sign the papers to take the drugs?" Tom Sell remembered being so cold he was shaking, and eventually the nurse warned that the stress would kill him and he was released from his shackles and returned to his cell. A week later, Dr. Sell's wrists were still cut, and his hands, arms, and legs were severely bruised. Dr. DeMier allegedly told Sell that "things will only get worse for you now."

In addition to the video camera that one of the guards had when Dr. Sell was removed from his cell, there were video cameras present in the cell where he was chained. Tom Sell's brother, Mark Sell, filed a complaint in January 2000 with Missouri Senators Christopher Bond (R-MO), John Ashcroft (R-MO) and U.S. Representative Jim Talent (R-MO) requesting a Congressional inquiry into the mistreatment of Tom Sell. Indeed, several more Republican Congress members representing Missouri also signed written requests for a federal investigation of Tom Sell's treatment.

Mark Sell also requested a copy of the videos recording the shackling incident. On May 4, 2000, Senators Bond and Ashcroft requested that Springfield prison furnish the video tapes and information relating to the November 9 incident. After numerous appeals through the Freedom of Information Act, the Bureau of Prisons informed Mark Sell on September 19, 2000, that no information exists on the incident.

The Bureau of Prison's claim, however, was disputed by Dennis Bitz, an attorney for the U.S. Department of Justice and Federal Bureau of Prisons. Bitz declared that he was aware of two investigation files pertaining to a "calculated use of force episode that allegedly occurred on November 9, 1999." The files were numbered SPGU-218-00 and SPGU-183-99. There was also a videotape file numbered SPG-00-007.[48] These files and tapes have never been released.

A front-page story in the *Post-Dispatch* in September 2001 prompted Senator John Ashcroft to meet with two local supporters of Dr. Tom Sell— Mark Sell and Thomas Bugel. The meeting lasted 10 minutes and was held at the airport in Saint Louis.

The media immediately focused upon Ashcroft's meeting to discuss the plight of Dr. Sell. They accused him of hypocrisy for being a "law and or-der" advocate and yet intervening on behalf of a white criminal defendant that is supported by the CCC. At the time, Ashcroft was undergoing Senate confirmation for the post of Attorney General.

A major point of opposition to his confirmation was his alleged racial bias in the confirmation hearings of Ronnie White to a federal judgeship on the grounds that the black jurist was "pro-criminal." The press immediately seized upon Ashcroft's support in the Sell case and implied that he was a supporter of the CCC. Dr. Sell's position is that the entire government case against him is meritless. He is perfectly sane and is entitled to a public trial to prove his innocence. When a defendant says he is sane and wants a trial, how can the government avoid a trial by claiming the defendant is not sane? Perhaps this is the new government strategy when it has a weak case.

Many observers believed that the government was retaliating against Dr. Sell's speaking out about his role in Waco, where he was summoned to do forensic dental analysis on the eve of the final raid on the Davidian compound. Dr. Sell said that he saw the FBI siege end on closed-circuit tele-vision. If true, the Department of Justice was likely to maintain the status quo by imprisoning Dr. Sell for years longer.

Justifying Forced Medication

In March 2002, the Eight Circuit Court of Appeals overturned the lower court's finding that Dr. Sell was dangerous. However, by a vote of 2-1, they found that "charges of fraud" alone are "serious" enough to justify forced medication. They also held that there are no limits on the quantity or type of drugs. The state had the power to inject Dr. Tom Sell forcibly with any drugs to make him mentally fit for trial.

This means that the government could force a citizen to take dangerous mind-altering drugs before a trial is even held. The ruling set off alarm bells in the civil liberties community. Civil libertarians feared that the Sell case would set a dangerous precedent. They argued that the use of powerful and untested drugs violated the Nuremberg Code, which bars using such drugs on prisoners.

On appeal, the U.S. Supreme Court handed down a 6-3 decision on the Sell case in July 2003 (Sell v. United States, No. 02-5664). They overturned the 8th Circuit Court ruling that permitted the forced medication of Dr. Sell.

The court set out a four-point test that the federal government must meet before imposing involuntary medication on a nonviolent prisoner awaiting trial: alternative treatment must be offered, the drug is likely to work, it is medically appropriate, and the defendant must have committed a serious crime.

This ruling did not resolve Dr. Sell's legal nightmare, however. Writing for the majority, Justice Stephen G. Breyer commented that Dr. Sell had already spent as long in prison as his sentence would be if he were convicted of the crimes of which he was accused. In a dissenting opinion, Justice Antonin Scalia objected that Dr. Sell's trial should have gone forward and the objection to forced medication postponed till after a conviction.

On April 15, 2005, Dr. Sell finally accepted the government's offer of "nolo contendere" or no contest and pled guilty to one count of fraud and one count of murder conspiracy in order to gain his freedom. He was released from jail the same day and was order to spend six months in a halfway house followed by three years of parole. He had lost his dental business, retirement funds, and his home. This ended the longest period of incarceration of an American citizen without a trial in the country's history.

6

PROSECUTORIAL OVERREACH: ANTI-KICKBACK LAWS AND THE "PINELLAS 14"

Another prosecutorial trap for doctors is the so-called Anti-Kickback Laws. These laws have criminalized doctors' referrals of patients to laboratories, clinics, hospitals, and medical supply companies in which they have a financial interest. Even though doctors are allowed to own their practices and receive payments from outside companies, they are subject to civil and criminal penalties for unintentionally referring patients to fraudulent firms.[1]

The laws are so ambiguous and contradictory that any ambitious U.S. Attorney can use them to destroy the careers and families of outstanding physicians who have dedicated their lives to the care of patients. Based upon testimony of confessed criminals and flawed documents, doctors have been arrested, indicted, convicted, and sentenced to prison. This happened to 14 doctors in West Florida in 2000.

A POLITICALLY AMBITIOUS U.S. ATTORNEY

Gary Montilla was an ambitious 50-year-old Assistant U.S. Attorney in the Middle District of Florida at the time of the prosecution. He was educated in Puerto Rico and was a private attorney in San Juan. Montilla became Puerto Rico's district director for the U.S. Census in 1979 and chief of the civil division of the Office of the U.S. Attorney in Puerto Rico from 1980 to 1986. His lifelong ambition was to become Puerto Rico's U.S. Attorney.

In 1995, Montilla took charge of a federal antifraud program called Operation Restore Trust (ORT) in the Tampa Bay area of West Florida. The purpose of ORT was to "fight fraud, waste and abuse" in the Medicare and Medicaid programs. The initial focus of the antifraud initiative was five states that had more than a third of all Medicare and Medicaid beneficiaries. These states were California, Florida, Illinois, New York, and Texas. Tampa Bay, Florida, had one of the highest per capita Medicare populations in the entire country. It also had the reputation for being a hotbed of scam artists and corrupt businesses preying upon the elderly.

From 1998–1999, only 52 physicians in the country were indicted and tried for fraudulently billing Medicare. In every case the doctors directly billed Medicare. Montilla sought to advance his professional career by leading all U.S. Attorneys in the country in health fraud prosecutions. His investigations were highly successful, and he was responsible for about 10 percent of all kickback health fraud cases in the entire country. He was credited with collecting more than $15 million in fines, forfeitures, and restitutions.

Montilla pioneered a prosecutorial method that became a model for health care investigators throughout the country. His new model for fraud prosecutions focused upon doctors whom he claimed "get rich on a steady diet of kickbacks."[2] Montilla said, "I know of physicians who are making upwards of $7,000 to $8,000 a month who never see a patient." He developed a streamlined prosecutorial method that he called "a blue-collar approach to white-collar crime."[3]

He said that the principal obstacles to health care prosecutions were patient confidentiality and proving that medical procedures were not "medically necessary." Montilla got around these barriers by simply following the money. He traced the checks issued by fraudulent medical companies to physicians who referred patients to them for laboratory tests, therapy, and supplies. In Montilla's mind, any doctor who received such payments had violated Anti-Kickback Laws whether they were aware of the fraud or not. To get convictions, Montilla did not have to worry about getting patients to testify against their doctors, prove that patient referrals were not medically necessary or that doctors had fraudulently billed the government. Montilla described it as a "nuts-and-bolts approach." "It's a way to get at the bad apples, which is economical, quick and efficient."[4] In other words, Montilla's new strategy was to indict and prosecute doctors who unknowingly received payment for services rendered to a private laboratory, clinic, or medical firm that committed fraud.

In 1998, Montilla was given the prestigious National Prosecutorial Award by the Federal Law Enforcement Officer's Association. He said, "I've become fascinated with health care fraud, I think it is going to be with us forever."[5]

MONTILLA TARGETS 400 DOCTORS

In 1998, Montilla described an ambitious plan he had to investigate and prosecute hundreds of doctors.[6] He said that he was going to investigate 400 physicians in the Tampa Bay area for illegal patient referrals to a fraudulent laboratory called the Clearwater Clinical Laboratory (CCL).

CCL was established in 1957 by James McKeown, Sr., who built the lab into one of Florida's largest privately owned medical labs with 150 employees. His son, James McKeown, Jr., took over the day-to-day operations of CCL in the 1990s and earned an estimated $800,000 as the vice president and director of marketing. About 1,200 doctors in Pinellas, Pasco, and Hernando countries sent blood and urine samples to CCL for testing.

Montilla went after 400 doctors whom Montilla said took money from CCL in exchange for sending their elderly patients' blood work there. The lab billed Medicare for the cost of doing the tests. Gary Montilla expected to convict 100 doctors for criminal fraud and convict another 100 doctors for civil fraud. An additional 100 physicians would have to repay the government for improper payments from CCL. Montilla was trying to set a national precedent that would enable the government to charge doctors for sending patients to laboratories that overbilled Medicare. From Montilla's point of view, this was a spectacular opportunity to make a mark for himself, and it was a financial bonanza for the government.

Montilla's strategy to target physicians for prosecution began in June 1998. The FBI served search warrants upon CCL's offices and seized boxes of financial records and contracts with doctors as part of its investigation into allegations of Medicare kickback fraud. One FBI agent described CCL as the largest payer of illegal kickbacks in the area. He said that 60 percent of the lab's business was Medicare billings and that CCL received $6.5 million from Medicare in 1977 alone.[7]

These documents formed the basis of what Montilla called the "top 20" list of doctors receiving CCL kickbacks. Five of the 20 physicians were the first to be indicted in Montilla's grandiose scheme to convict hundreds of doctors. He subsequently indicted a total of 14 doctors in the Tampa area for allegedly steering $1.4 million in Medicare business to CCL in exchange for $400,000 in kickbacks. These doctors were dubbed the "Pinellas 14" by the media after Pinellas County, Florida. Montilla correctly reasoned that if he could convict the top "kickback recipients," other doctors would quickly fall into line and plead guilty in order to avoid the public humiliation and ruin of a trial.

The alleged kickbacks were CCL payments to physicians for personal service contracts called Medical and Technical Review Officers (MROs and TROs). Doctors who signed MRO contracts were supposed to review test reports in the CCL labs of their offices, and TROs were supposed to authorize patients to have CCL lab tests if their doctors were not available. According to prosecutors, CCL's most common kickbacks were for "do-nothing jobs" as technical consultants or for overly generous rents for space and equipment in physicians' offices.[8]

Montilla ordered secret FBI-taped conversations between Jason Welles, a CCL sales representative and FBI informant, and his CCL boss, Vincent Gepp.[9] Gepp was initially hired by CCL as a sales representative in 1995 and became the general manager of the company in 1997. Gepp never finished high school but by 1998 he was making a $100,000. During the trial, Gepp was asked why he participated in the fraud conspiracy. He said, "I have a wife and two kids and with that education where could I get another job for $100,000 a year. I can give you 100,000 reasons why I participated in the fraud."[10]

The conversations between Welles and Gepp were taped between February and March 1998 and were staged by Welles and the FBI. When Gepp and the father and son owners of CCL, James McKeown, Sr., and James McKeown, Jr., were presented with the FBI tapes, they agreed to plead guilty and attempted to transfer guilt for the conspiracy to the doctors. They told the FBI that the contracts they signed with the doctors were sham agreements designed to obtain fraudulent referrals from the doctors. Vincent Gepp made contemptuous statements about the doctors.

For example, on March 3, 1998, Gepp said if CCL pays doctors $500 a month to rent their office space, the lab can get "a big fat sloppy bastard" to refer patients to CCL.[11] Gepp elaborated on the theme of greedy physicians:

> All doctors love cash. I've sat there and dropped an envelope with cashiers checks all through the fucking counter, bags of money.[12]

In 1995, there was a change in Medicare rules that led to CCL's fraud conspiracy. The change prohibited CCL from paying rent to doctors for the space they were using in their offices to conduct CCL blood tests. It also required that the phlebotomist (a technician who draws blood and urine samples) work only for CCL and not for the doctor.

This led Jim McKeown, Jr., and CCL's attorney Les Conkley to come up with the idea of a Technical Review Officer (TRO) and a Medical Review Officer (MRO) as a way to bribe doctors for CCL patient referrals. CCL stopped paying doctors for renting space in their offices, but continued to pay them using the subterfuge of TROs or MROs service contracts.

Gepp testified that CCL used TRO positions as a way to bribe doctors for patients' laboratory referrals. He said that the conspiracy was created by McKeown, Jr., and Les Conklin. When a doctor's referrals to CCL dropped below an acceptable level, the doctor would be removed from CCL's TRO program and the monthly payments to him would stop. Gepp stated that the doctors were very naive and believed everything they were told about the TRO payments.[13] Gepp said that Dr. Michael Peter Spuza, one of the doctors who was later prosecuted, was an idiot when it came to business, and he did not pay attention at business meetings.

Montilla presented this information to a federal grand jury in Tampa in late 1998. In early 1999, the grand jury returned a 68-count indictment against Vincent Gepp, James McKeown, Sr., James McKeown, Jr., and five doctors. The indictment charged the defendants with Medicare fraud, kickbacks, and conspiracy.

THE DOCTORS AS SCAPEGOATS

Montilla subsequently dropped the 28 felony counts against the CCL executives in exchange for their cooperation in the case against the doctors—the real target of the investigation. Gepp and McKeown, Sr., were given three years' probation without making any monetary repayment to Medicare. James McKeown, Jr., received a sentence of six months in a halfway house because of his involvement in an unrelated insurance fraud in the scuttling of his yacht. None of the three executives were fined.

Incredulously, the McKeowns were allowed to keep $2.5 million they defrauded from the government and were even permitted to sell the company's assets to another lab called Med-Tech. The sale occurred in August 1998, after the FBI seized CCL's files and started criminal investigations of the company. Hence, Gepp and the McKeowns were allowed to continue receiving fraudulent laboratory profits from Medicare during two years of the investigation.

James McKeown, Jr., also received $16,000 a month in sales-rental payments during these years; and Gepp became the president of the new company Med-Tech. Gepp acquired 25 percent ownership of its stock and continued operating the lab, billing Medicare, and received a monthly salary of $10,000 for 18 months after the FBI's seizure of CCL's records.

By contrast, there was no plea bargain for the doctors. Montilla targeted 5 physicians on his list of 20 kickback recipients for prosecution. They were Russell Charles Bufalino, 62; Robert L. Hartzell, 41; Ira Harvey Liss, 53; Cesar A. Lara, 43; and Michael Peter Spuza, 40. The physicians were charged with receiving kickbacks from CCL in the amount of $28,000, $27,000, $8,100, $32,000, and $12,000, respectively.

After they were charged, the doctors received a call from the Marshall's office and were told to report by 1:00 P.M. or they would become fugitives. None of the doctors had ever been investigated or indicted for any offense. They were family and primary care physicians who, for the most part, did not even know one another.

Nevertheless, they were arrested and paraded through the streets of Tampa in handcuffs. They were shackled at the ankles on a bench and held in a jail cell for six hours until the bond hearing before a federal judge. Unlike the CCL executives, all Medicare payments for the services that the doctors had already rendered were immediately suspended without notice or appeal. Since most of the doctors were heavily dependent upon Medicare payments, this virtually assured their bankruptcy.

"SPOKE AND WHEEL": A FALSE ANALOGY

Montilla used the analogy of a spoke and wheel to incriminate the doctors in an alleged conspiracy to defraud the government. He argued before the jury that CCL was the hub and the doctors were the spokes of the wheel.

The so-called kickbacks were CCL payments to doctors for supervising the operation of their labs, called draw stations, and evaluating the test results. CCL paid the physicians between a few hundred dollars and $1,500 per month to serve as MROs and TROs. Montilla used the testimony of Gepp and the McKeowns to argue to the jury that MRO and TRO payments to doctors violated the Anti-Kickback Laws and made them guilty of conspiracy to defraud Medicare. Since the "hub" of the conspiracy, CCL, had already pled guilty to the fraud conspiracy, what remained was to convict the "spokes" of the wheel conspiracy—the doctors.

The analogy was false, however. In order for a wheel conspiracy to exist, the people who form the wheel's spokes must be aware of each other and must do something to advance a single, illegal action. Otherwise, the alleged conspiracy lacks "the rim of the wheel to enclose the spokes."[14] Most of the 14 physicians who were indicted for conspiracy did not know one another. None of them had any knowledge of the others' business. None of them had conspiratorial information to provide the government.

Until CCL was raided by the FBI in 1998, the physicians had no idea that there was a conspiracy to defraud the government. CCL had been in business in the Tampa Bay area for 40 years and had an excellent reputation in the medical community for prompt turnaround time and accurate test results. The doctors had no reason to question the legality of dealing with CCL. Attorneys assured the doctors that the contracts with CCL were legitimate.[15]

CCL's lawyers, Conklin & Sauey, supplied the doctors with an opinion letter in March 1994. The letter declared that CCL's MRO and TRO contracts with the doctors satisfied the "safe harbor" exemption to the Anti-Kickback Laws.[16] Many of the doctors also consulted their own attorneys about the legality of the contracts. For example, Dr. Michael Spuza's attorney, Lucas Selly, examined the CCL contracts and advised Dr. Spuza that they were legal.

THE DOCTORS' TRIAL

In April 2000, Montilla prosecuted what he called the ringleaders of the doctors' kickback conspiracy in order to intimidate other physicians into pleading guilty to fraud. They were Dr. Michael Spuza and Dr. Ira Harvey Liss. They had never met until they were arrested.

Drs. Spuza and Liss were tried at the same time and were each charged with one count of conspiring to defraud the Medicare program and five counts of receiving illegal kickbacks. The allegation was that CCL paid Spuza $12,000 for patient referrals while receiving $269,000 in Medicare reimbursements. Dr. Liss was charged with receiving $29,000 from CCL in exchange for referring $183,847 in Medicare payments to CCL. Each doctor faced a maximum penalty of 30 years in prison and a $1.5 million fine.

The heart of the government's case against Spuza and Liss was their alleged "corrupt intentions" in referring patients to CCL. The doctors did not dispute the payments they received from CCL, and the government did not question the legality of the contracts CCL signed with the physicians. The basis of the doctors' alleged kickback conspiracy was that money flowed from CCL to the physicians and that the doctors did nothing in return for it.

The government's proof of the doctors' corrupt intentions was the testimony of CCL's executives, owners, and sales staff. The prosecution's chief witness in the trial was Vincent Gepp, CCL's general manager. Gepp testified that the doctors helped CCL defraud Medicare alone out of more than $2 million a year. The guilt or innocence of the doctors was largely based upon the truthfulness of Gepp's testimony.

Vincent Gepp and the McKeowns pled guilty to Medicare fraud in April 2000, just before the trial began. This raises questions about the credibility of their testimony. They had a powerful incentive to implicate the doctors in Montilla's plan to convict hundreds of physicians for receiving kickbacks from CCL. For example, in response to questions about CCL's relationship with Dr. Spuza, Vincent Gepp said, "If renting the equipment and space did not convince Dr. Spuza to send laboratory work to our lab, we would offer to provide Test Review Officer (TRO) compensation and see if that would get him to commit to CCL."[17] Gepp insisted that Dr. Spuza's appointment as a TRO was a carrot to win his business.[18]

On cross-examination, Gepp contradicted his testimony, however. On the one hand, he said that Dr. Spuza did not provide services for the TRO contract. On the other hand, he acknowledged that Dr. Spuza did "arterial sticks" in the CCL lab of his office. Drawing blood from a patient's artery instead of a vein is more difficult and is usually done by doctors. Gepp also acknowledged that Dr. Spuza authorized and reviewed CCL lab test results.[19]

> If a patient from New York or New Jersey showed up at the draw station, we would draw the blood and Dr. Spuza would look at the results because there is no local doctor.[20]

The defense asked Gepp if Dr. Spuza billed for that service and Gepp said, "No, that would be what the TRO fee would be for."[21] Incredulously, Gepp maintained that Dr. Spuza did nothing for CCL.

The phlebotomist who drew blood at CCL's draw station in Dr. Spuza's clinic, Efrain Arrazola, supported Michael Spuza's defense. Arrazola said that Dr. Spuza checked CCL's lab reports everyday—sometimes twice a day. Arrazola said that when he had a hard time with a patient, when patients lost consciousness, when there were difficulties drawing blood, or when he needed help complying with the government's Occupational Safety Health Regulations (OSHA) regulations, Dr. Spuza assisted him.[22]

CCL CONSPIRACY EXCLUDED FROM TRIAL

The government acknowledged that CCL was guilty of two fraudulent Medicare billing conspiracies. The first was "unbundling." Unbundling occurs when a doctor orders a set of tests (called a panel) for a general evaluation of a patient and CCL breaks the panel into two different sets of tests for billing purposes. By billing Medicare for two sets of six tests instead of a panel of 12 tests, CCL was able to increase the Medicare payment from $25 to $47. On average, CCL billed Medicare between 50 and 130 percent more for the tests than they were legally entitled.

The second fraudulent scheme was that CCL billed for tests such as cholesterol, iron, or blood sugar that were never requested by a physician. The CCL would not actually perform the tests but would bill Medicare for them, using the doctors' names. The physicians were not aware that their names were used by CCL to bill Medicare for nonexistent tests. The magnitude or frequency of CCL's fraudulent billing was never investigated by the government, and the amount of the fraud was never calculated. It was conservatively estimated by the defense to be at least $15 million.

The doctors' alleged guilt in the CCL conspiracy was distorted and exaggerated because CCL's crime was barred from the trial. After CCL executives pled guilty to fraud, Montilla placed the full weight of the conspiracy upon the doctors. Without exposing CCL's plot, it was impossible to clear the physicians of the charges. In other words, in order to explain to the jury that the doctors were innocent pawns in CCL's conspiracy to defraud Medicare, they had to expose the real perpetrators of the crime—CCL executives.

Gepp and the McKeown could not be cross-examined at the trial about the CCL fraud. The judge did not even allow the defense to question CCL officials about the conspiracy. James McKeown, Jr., avoided testimony altogether by invoking his Fifth Amendment rights against self-incrimination. Every attempt by the defense to expose CCL's conspiracy was deflected by Montilla who simply said that "CCL pled guilty already; they're not on trial."[23]

If the defense had been able to expose CCL's criminal conspiracy, they would have been able to cast doubt upon the credibility of the government's witnesses. Gepp's trustworthiness was already in doubt because of his involvement in an unrelated criminal conspiracy.

Vincent Gepp and Jim McKeown, Jr., were involved in an insurance fraud conspiracy to sink McKeown's 46-foot boat, the *Marlintini*, valued at $250,000. The yacht was docked at his palatial home in Seminole, Florida. McKeown, Jr., gave Gepp $5,000 to pay a man to take the *Marlintini* out to sea and sink it by shooting holes in the hull with a shotgun and handgun. McKeown could not afford to keep the boat but could not sell it. Montilla granted Gepp immunity from prosecution for this conspiracy in exchange for his testimony against the doctors.

U.S. District Judge Richard A. Lazzara, the judge in the case, also imposed the "one purpose" rule at trial. This virtually guaranteed the doctors' conviction. The rule is that if one purpose of the money the doctors received from CCL was to induce the referral of Medicare business, they must be found guilty of violating the Anti-Kickback Laws. This rule applies regardless of the percentage of money that financially benefited the physicians. For example, if only 1 percent of the payments by CCL financially benefited the doctors, they are guilty of fraud.

This ruling completely overturned the "safe harbors" exemption to the Anti-Kickback Laws. If a doctor unknowingly received payments from a fraudulent company to which they send Medicare patients, they have violated the Anti-Kickback Laws and there are no defenses against it.

The "Ebb and Flow" Theory

In addition to Gepp's self-serving testimony, Montilla introduced misleading evidence of the doctors' alleged conspiracy. Gary Montilla presented what he called an "ebb and flow" theory of kickbacks as the linchpin of his case. In his opening statement at the trial, Montilla said that he would provide evidence that would prove the "ebb and flow" of kickbacks to Drs. Spuza and Liss.

Montilla argued that "when there was money, patients were referred to CCL and when there wasn't any money, the patients stopped."[24] In other words, when the money flowed from CCL to the doctors, the patients flowed from the doctors to CCL, and when the money stopped, the patients stopped going to CCL.

In Montilla's closing statement to the jury, he said that in the summer of 1996 Dr. Spuza had a dispute with CCL and there was suddenly a "big dip" in Michael Spuza's patient referrals to CCL. Montilla explained it in the following way:

> Dr. Spuza took the hose of referrals that was flowing to CCL and doubled it up and stopped the referrals. He shut off the flow of patients because he was demanding more money from CCL. Once he got the agreement he wanted with CCL, he strung out the hose and opened the flow of referrals to the lab.[25]

Gary Montilla asked Lorraine Watson, a senior fraud investigator for the insurance company that processed Medicare payments in West Florida, to analyze the doctors' "patient referrals" from 1995 through 1998. Watson erroneously testified in the trial that she counted the doctors' patient referrals to CCL from 1995 to 1998.

In fact, what she actually counted was bills submitted by CCL to Medicare, which included fraudulent laboratory services. Gary Montilla used this information instead of the physicians' actual patient referrals to CCL at the trial. He presented the information in Column C of Table 6.1 to support his ebb and flow theory as applied to Dr. Spuza.

According to Montilla, Dr. Spuza had a dispute with Gepp and McKeown, Jr., over the amount of money they were paying him, and he stopped referring patients to CCL in June and July of 1996 as a way of exerting leverage to extract more money from CCL. After CCL agreed to Dr. Spuza's financial demands, the flow of patient referrals resumed in August 1996. Likewise, after CCL payments for Spuza's TRO appointment ended in July 1998, Dr. Spuza allegedly stopped his referrals to CCL. Similarly, after CCL cancelled Dr. Liss's TRO, he allegedly stopped sending patients to the lab.

Contrary to Montilla's claims, not only was the data he presented to the jury erroneous, but, in fact, there was no ebb and flow in Dr. Spuza's or Dr. Liss's patient referrals to CCL at all. According to Dr. Spuza's office records, he referred 29 patients to CCL for blood work in 1995, 57 in 1996, and 107 in 1997, and 213 in 1998. In fact, Spuza referred patients to CCL every

Table 6.1
Spuza's Records and CCL Billing Fraud

	Michael Spuza's Actual Patient Referrals[a]	CCL Billing for Spuza's Patients[b]	CCL Billing for Spuza's Lab[c]
1996			
January	3	144	921
February	4	169	886
March	7	144	583
April	3	85	127
May	3	131	133
June	2	13	14
July	1	1	1
August	9	51	573
September	13	123	560
October	6	44	595
November	4	25	575
December	2	11	157
Total	*57*	*941*	*5,125*
1998			
January	10	128	872
February	13	129	649
March	16	190	662
April	16	351	1048
May	31	442	1189
June	21	278	904
July	4	50	149
August	49	0	0
September	17	0	0
October	18	0	0
November	18	0	0
December	0	0	0
Total	*213*	*1,568*	*5,473*

Note: [a]Dr. Michael Spuza's office patient referrals based upon laboratory requisition forms in the Spuza Clinic. Data compiled by Christie Nicholas, R.N.

[b]Summary of lab tests CCL billed Medicare in the name of Dr. Michael Spuza. Data compiled by Lorraine Watson, Senior Fraud Investigator for First Coast Options, the Florida Medicare insurance carrier intermediary.

[c]Summary of lab tests CCL billed Medicare in the names of Dr. Michael Spuza and Dr. Felicia Spuza. Data compiled by Lorraine Watson. Gary Montilla introduced this to the jury at the trial of Dr. Spuza and Dr. Liss in April 2000.

month during 1996, 1997, and 1998. Gary Montilla's claim that there was a "big dip" in Dr. Spuza's CCL referrals during the summer of 1996 was an illusion.

CCL's Billing Fraud

The doctors' defense lawyers were not given the CCL's Medicare billing records. They did not have an opportunity to prepare an adequate response to it. After the trial, they did examine the data presented by the government and compared it to Dr. Spuza's office patient records. They found major discrepancies between the data that Montilla presented to the jury and Dr. Spuza's patient referral records. It was impossible to reconcile the two.

In the first place, the government's evidence of Dr. Spuza's fraudulent referrals (Table 6.1 Column C) was not Michael Spuza's patient referrals to CCL. It was the number of laboratory tests that CCL billed Medicare. Since CCL pled guilty to fraudulently billing Medicare, the services that they billed Medicare in Dr. Spuza's name inflated the actual number of tests that Michael Spuza's ordered for patients. There was no way of knowing how many lab tests Dr. Spuza ordered for his patients except to examine his office records.

Christie Nichols, Michael Spuza's nurse, companion, and office manager from October 1996 to April 1997, painstakingly searched thousands of patient records in Dr. Spuza's office looking for the number of patient referrals that Dr. Spuza sent to CCL. She compared the number of patient referrals for lab tests that Dr. Spuza made (Table 6.1 Column A) with the number of services CCL billed Medicare in Dr. Spuza's name (Table 6.1 Columns B and C) in 1996 and 1998. For example, according to Dr. Spuza's office records, Michael Spuza referred only three patients to CCL in January of 1996. According to Medicare's records, CCL billed Medicare for 144 tests for the three patients Dr. Spuza referred to CCL that month. This works out to 48 separate blood tests per patient in one month; highly improbable. Furthermore, the government claimed that CCL billed Medicare in Dr. Spuza's name for a total of 921 lab tests (Table 6.1 Column C). According to Medicare, these bills were for CCL lab tests ordered by Dr. Michael Spuza and his mother, Dr. Felicia Spuza, with whom he practiced. In fact, there were at least 40 other doctors who referred patients to the CCL lab in Dr. Spuza's office. To argue that Dr. Spuza "steered" all of these referrals to CCL strains belief.

Table 6.1 (Column A) also shows that during the summer of 1996 and after July 1998, there was no ebb and flow in Dr. Spuza's patient referrals. In fact, Michael Spuza never stopped referring patients to CCL (see Table 6.1 Column A). This is despite the fact that Dr. Spuza replaced CCL with another lab in his clinic from January to August 1996. Contrary to the government's claim, Dr. Spuza did not stop referring patients to CCL after July 1998.

In August 1998, Dr. Spuza referred 49 patients, in September 17 patients, October 18 patients, and November 18 patients. If there was any fluctuation in patient referrals, it was the arrival and departure of retired "snow birds" from the north who migrated to Florida for the summer and return after September each year.

Using the fraudulent CCL Medicare bills (Table 6.1 Column C), Gary Montilla characterized Dr. Spuza as a ringleader of the doctors' conspiracy. In fact, Michael Spuza had no control over other doctor's referrals to CCL. CCL's draw station in Dr. Spuza's clinic was open to the public. Anyone could go to the lab for a blood or urine test.

The fraud investigator listed Michael Spuza on all Medicare bills as the requisitioning doctor for patients sent to the lab in his clinic. The reason for this is that Michael Spuza was one of Vincent Gepp's clients. As Gepp's physician-client, Vincent Gepp programmed the computer in Dr. Spuza's CCL lab to automatically list Michael Spuza as the doctor requisitioning all lab tests. This was without regard for which doctor actually referred the patient to the lab. Gepp did this to ensure that he received his 3 percent commission of income derived from all patients referred to Dr. Spuza's draw station.

DESTRUCTION OF DOCTORS' CAREERS

Based upon the self-serving testimony of confessed criminals and bogus data, Dr. Spuza and Dr. Liss were convicted on all counts and were given prison sentences. The sentences were based upon the dollar amount of the fraud plus "enhancements" for being doctors and violating the "trust of Medicare." The judge added CCL's office rent and equipment sublease payments to the $12,000 paid to Dr. Spuza for a combined "kickback" of $55,371.36. He did this despite the fact that none of the rental or lease money ever passed through Dr. Spuza's hands. Furthermore, the leases were not even in his name. They were in Dr. Felicia Spuza's name.

Dr. Liss received a prison sentence of 15 months for kickbacks in the amount of $29,000, plus breach of trust of Medicare and obstruction of justice. The doctors lost their medical licenses, their practices, their homes, and were forced to declare bankruptcy. Dr. Spuza spent more than $300,000 in legal fees attempting to defend himself.

This case devastated the medical community in Tampa Bay. The doctors were sent to prison despite the fact that they were not guilty of unnecessary testing, harming patients, or fraudulently billing the government. Many believed that they were only guilty of being naive and believing the lies of criminal businessmen who were on the fringes of medicine and whose only interest was making money.

The case set a dangerous precedent that enables the government to criminally prosecute doctors in cases where they send patients to labs that overbill Medicare. Twelve additional physicians who faced similar charges accepted plea agreements rather than take their chances in court.

Dr. Randy A. Shuck explained the impact that the case had upon the physicians. Based upon 2 convictions, 12 indicted doctors were goaded into accepting pleas with the government that effectively ended their medical careers.

They were stripped of their dignity, were financially bankrupted, and embarrassed publicly.

Tampa Bay has had the greatest number of kickback fraud investigations in the country. This was largely due to a politically ambitious prosecuting attorney who ignored the real criminals behind a multimillion-dollar Medicare fraud conspiracy schemes. Instead, the prosecutor targeted naïve family physicians who unknowingly received modest payments from a corrupt laboratory in order to gain national publicity and celebrity recognition associated with prosecuting a large number of doctors. Montilla justified his strategy by "scaring the doctors straight."[26]

Montilla's political stock rose dramatically after his conviction of the doctors. In 2001, Gary Montilla was nominated by President Bush to become the new U.S. attorney for Puerto Rico, thus fulfilling his lifetime ambition. The "Pinellas 14" doctors, the Tampa Bay medical community, and thousands of patients were not so fortunate, however. The ambition of a single prosecutor destroyed the careers and lives of more than a dozen doctors and their families. Their exclusion from Medicare will cause the entire health care system in West Florida to suffer. The core of family doctors who are the main medical resource of the elderly population there is now in jeopardy.

7

DEA Drug Warriors: Targeting Doctors as Drug Dealers

According to the government, a small group of doctors prescribe hundreds of millions of dollars of dangerous narcotics that feed a booming black market of illegal drugs and contribute to an epidemic of addiction, crime, and death.[1] Hollywood has provided prosecutors with a stereotypical image of a narcissistic drug-addicted doctor in the hit television series, *House, M.D.* Dr. House is portrayed as a brilliant but unstable drug-addicted physician who is antisocial and rebellious and defies drug laws. This provides the societal backdrop for prosecuting physicians.

Indeed, doctors have been tried as drug kingpins and dealers for manslaughter in the deaths of pain patients who misused and overdosed on drugs they were prescribed. When convicted, physicians are subject to the same draconian mandatory drug sentencing guidelines that were designed to punish violent, illegal drug dealers.

The sentences for these physicians are based upon the number and weight of pills that they prescribe to patients. These highly publicized indictments and prosecutions have intimidated many physicians out of pain management, leaving only a few thousand doctors in the country who are still willing to risk prosecution and ruin in order to treat patients who are suffering from severe chronic pain. In Florida, for example, the fourth most populous state, only 1 percent, or 574 of the state's 56,926 doctors, prescribed the vast majority of narcotic drugs paid for by Medicaid in 2003.[2]

Dr. J. David Haddox, the vice president of health affairs at Purdue Pharma L.D., the manufacturer of OxyContin and MSContin, long-acting opioid pain relieving medications, estimates that there are between 4,000 or 5,000 doctors specialized in pain management in the entire country to treat at least 30 million chronic pain sufferers.[3] Or, to put it another way, there is just 1 pain doctor for 6,000 chronic pain patients in need of treatment.

Pain patients can suffer from a wide range of illnesses and disabilities, including lower back pain, rheumatoid arthritis, shingles, postsurgical pain, fibromyalgia, sickle cell anemia, diabetes, HIV/AIDS, migraine and cluster headaches, pain from broken bones, sports injuries, and other trauma. According to the American Pain Foundation, over 75 million Americans suffer from serious pain each year, 50 million of them from serious chronic pain (lasting six months or more), and an additional 25 million endure acute pain from accidents, surgeries, and injuries. In a survey conducted in 1999, only one in four with pain receives adequate treatment.[4] One study of children who died from cancer at two Boston hospitals between 1990 and 1997 found that almost 90 percent of them had "substantial suffering in the last month and attempts to control their symptoms were often unsuccessful."[5]

Since pain is the principal reason that patients seek medical care, the prosecution of doctors who treat chronic pain has added to an already-serious health problem in the country—the undertreatment of pain. The societal cost of pain sufferers is enormous. In addition to the obvious cost of needless suffering, it also includes broken marriages, alcoholism and family violence, absenteeism and job loss, depression, and suicide. The American Pain Society estimated that in 1995, untreated pain cost American business over $100 billion a year in medical expenses, lost wages, and other costs plus the loss of 50 million workdays.[6]

DRUG TOLERANCE AND INTOLERANCE

The United States has historically wavered between eras of drug tolerance and eras of intolerance. Familiarity with that history helps put the current war on pain doctors into perspective. The targeting of physicians is nothing new. During periods of extreme drug intolerance, the government has frequently targeted doctors in its quixotic quest to eradicate drug addiction.

According to Yale University's David Musto, the United States has gone through several historical periods of drug tolerance and intolerance.[7] These periods roughly correspond to swings in the public's attitude toward other addictive substances, notably alcohol and tobacco. The periods of general drug tolerance were from the 1880s to 1914, and from the 1960s to 1980. The periods of drug intolerance took place from 1920 (the adoption of Prohibition) to 1933, and from 1981 to the present. These swings in the public attitude toward drugs are due in large part to the societal fear of addiction, which tends to rise during the public's awareness of dangerous drugs and heightened social and political hardships. Earlier periods of intolerance also show the same patterns of widespread public fear, media complicity, and government malevolence we see in the current war on opioids.

Drug Tolerance: The 1880s to 1914

From the introduction of heroin in the United States during the 1880s until Prohibition in 1920, narcotics were unregulated and widely available. Drug addiction was largely accidental, due to the public's ignorance about the habit-forming properties of the most popular highly addictive drug of the era, morphine. Though widely used for medical operations and convalescence, morphine was also used in everyday potions and elixirs.

The drug was commonly regarded as a universal panacea, used to treat as many as 54 diseases, ranging from insanity, diarrhea, dysentery, menstrual and menopausal pain, and nymphomania.[8] Opiates were as readily available in drug and grocery stores as aspirin is today. They served the same function that alcohol, tranquilizers, and antidepressants do today. Known to some physicians as "God's own medicine," morphine was a frequent additive to several household tonics and health elixirs. Potions such as "Doctor Smith's Tonic, Good for Man or Beast" were widely available in drugstores, and found in homes across the country. One company sold more than 600 drugs and other products containing opiates. For example, "Godfrey's Cordial" combined opium with molasses and sassafras for flavoring. This beverage was popular in the United States and Britain and was even given to infants under the age of two to soothe teething pain.

This widespread use of morphine, opium, and cocaine gave rise to between 250,000 and 1 million addicts in the United States out of a population of 76 million; a level of addiction never again reached. The typical addict between 1871 and 1922 was a middle-aged, rural, middle, or upper-middle class white housewife.[9] While social mores of the time discouraged women from imbibing alcohol, no such prohibition applied to opiates and many upper class women used the drugs for relaxation and relief from "women's troubles."

According to Dr. Charles E. Terry's popular 1914 book *The Opium Program*, 80 percent of all addicted patients treated in his public health clinic in Jacksonville, Florida, had jobs, homes, families, and "good reputations."[10] Addiction was not a reason for divorce and children were not taken from their parents and placed in foster homes when one or both parents were addicted. In other words, addicts continued to participate fully in society as good citizens. This situation changed dramatically when opiate addiction was criminalized and social stigma attached to users created a deviant subculture of addicts who were alienated from society.

Drug Intolerance, 1914–1933

Despite the fact that the affluent, reputable, and upper class were more prone to addiction than others, minority groups were quickly tagged as the stereotypical heroin and cocaine junkie, particularly black laborers in the south, and Chinese laborers on the west coast. By the time the Great Depression caused widespread unemployment, a growing resentment of cheap Chinese laborers took hold. And opium provided a convenient vehicle to villainize them.

William Randolph Hearst's tabloids, for example, began publishing sensational reports of "respectable white women" being seduced into "a life of prostitution and debauchery" in Chinese opium dens.[11] As for blacks, there were also widespread reports that construction companies in the South were supplying blacks with cocaine to boost labor output, and that the "cocaine-crazed Negro brain" was fueling an outbreak of attacks on white women.

During the "Red Scare" of the 1920s, public antidrug scorn turned to Bolsheviks and anarchists. Internal ethnic and racial groups already associated with drug addiction were linked to communism as well, and generally viewed as a threat to the moral strength of the nation.[12]

Despite the accidental nature of opium addiction, and that most addicts were white, and were productive members of society, the government embarked upon a draconian law enforcement policy designed to eradicate the scourge of addiction. The federal government profiled addicts as "criminal types" with weak moral character, who needed to be tracked down and isolated from society. The doctors who treated them were also targeted by law enforcement as the suppliers of narcotics to addicts. Thousands of doctors were prosecuted in this earliest effort to purge narcotics from common use.[13]

The Harrison Act

The first federal law to criminalize the nonmedical use of drugs was the Harrison Act of 1914, which criminalized the nonmedical use of opium, morphine, and cocaine.[14] The law was sponsored in large part by advocates of Prohibition.[15] Section 2 of the Act also made it illegal for any physician or druggist to prescribe narcotics to an addict, effectively turning a quarter of a million drug-addicted citizens and their doctors into criminals.[16]

In compliance with the Harrison Act, by 1916, 124,000 physicians, 47,000 druggists, 37,000 dentists, 11,000 veterinarians, and 1,600 manufacturers, wholesalers, and importers had registered with the Treasury Department.[17]

Almost as soon as they registered, hundreds of doctors were subsequently arrested and prosecuted for prescribing narcotics to addicted patients.[18] During the first 14 years of the Act, U.S. Attorneys prosecuted more than 77,000 violations, mostly medical professionals.[19] Between 1914 and 1938, about 25,000 doctors were arrested under the terms of the Harrison Act for giving narcotic prescriptions to addicts.[20] They were put on trial, and most lost their reputations, careers, and life savings. By 1928, the average sentence was 1 year and 10 months in prison.[21] More than 19 percent of all federal prisoners (2,529 of 7,738) were in prison for narcotics offenses.[22] Clinics closed down, and physicians had no choice but to abandon thousands of addicted patients. The United States quickly became the world's most lucrative market for underground narcotics.

On the eve of the repeal of Prohibition in 1932, the government called a halt to its persecution of doctors as a means of eradicating addiction. According to a high official of the Federal Bureau of Narcotics, Harry J. Anslinger, the commissioner of the Federal Bureau of Narcotics, announced that no federal agent could begin an investigation of a medical professional without written order from a supervisor. He felt that the day was over in which investigators "black-jack" (health professionals) into line.

Anslinger hoped to "eliminate the complaint on the part of some of the professional men against the desire of some of our field men to build up a good record at the expense of the professional classes, and made up a lot of petty cases which we didn't feel should be called to the attention of the United States Attorney, or even reported to the bureau cases that have merit." While the Harrison Act did not succeed in eradicating addiction, it did succeed in frightening doctors into refusing to treat addicted patients.[23]

Second Period of Drug Tolerance

From the repeal of Prohibition in 1933 to the end of the Carter administration, America coasted through a long spell of drug tolerance. The Pure Food and Drug Act of 1906 that required manufacturers to reveal the habit-forming properties of prescription drugs, helped to curb accidental addiction.[24] World War II disrupted the international flow of illegal narcotics, effectively drying up the domestic U.S. supply. The number of narcotics addicts dropped dramatically during the 1940s and 1950s and a new generation of Americans grew up without direct knowledge or fear of narcotics.

From 1960 to 1970, the country experienced unprecedented economic growth, including a doubling of the gross national product, with enough money in the treasury to wage both the Vietnam War and the War on Poverty. All of this wealth created an enormous demand for consumer goods and creature comforts. Extra wealth, the leisure time wealth frees up, and the sociocultural climate of the time led to a notable rise in the use of recreational drugs.

Yale's David Musto characterizes this period as the height of risk-taking in American culture. By the late 1960s, the Baby Boomer generation had entered its teen and young adulthood years (15–24), the age demographic most likely to experiment with drugs.[25] It was also the era of Woodstock, war protest, and countercultural attacks on traditional societal values. Cult figures such as Dr. Timothy Leary—who urged the young to "turn on, tune in, and drop out"—emerged, and won instant followings. In addition to heroin and marijuana, newer strains of drugs such as LSD and PCP grew popular.

The second era of U.S. drug tolerance hit its peak in 1978, when President Carter's head of drug policy in the White House, Dr. Peter G. Bourne, argued for decriminalizing marijuana. Bourne argued that marijuana wasn't comparably harmful, and inappropriately imprisoned a large number of middle-class youth. Bourne also argued that cocaine caused relatively few health and social consequences.[26]

Widespread use of illegal drugs became symbolic of 1960s youth rebellion and counterculture values, an association that's admittedly supported by statistics. Arrests by state law enforcement increased from 18,000 in 1965 to 188,000 in 1970. Narcotic-related hepatitis cases rose from 4,000 in 1966 to 36,000 in 1971, and heroin users increased from 50,000 in 1960 to more than 500,000 in 1970. The pendulum was set to swing the other way.

The Second Period of Drug Intolerance

The second period of drug intolerance began with the Reagan administration and continued through the Bush administration in 2007. In 1986, President and Mrs. Reagan repudiated the tolerant attitude toward drugs of the previous era. Nancy Reagan began a personal campaign against drugs, rousing support in the media by saying: "Each of us has a responsibility to be intolerant of drug use anywhere, any time, by anybody. We must create an atmosphere of intolerance for drug use in the country." Reagan invoked many of the same themes and metaphors of drug depravity, criminality, and threat to America's national security used during the first period of drug intolerance from 1914 to 1933.

Reagan announced the war on drugs shortly after the smokable form of cocaine crack appeared in certain parts of the country in 1985. The alleged crack epidemic created widespread fear. When the spread of AIDS hit the headlines, the one-two crack-AIDS punch set the stage for a massive public backlash against illicit drugs. In order to carry out the war on drugs, the administration enlisted the support of a powerful grassroots movement called the Parents' Movement. This was a nationwide movement of conservative parents' groups lobbying for stricter regulation of marijuana and the prevention of drug use by teenagers. With the support of the Drug Enforcement Agency (DEA) and the National Institute on Drug Abuse (NIDA), they were instrumental in fostering the changes in public attitudes necessary to mount the war on drugs.

In 1984, the Reagan administration sponsored the Federal Sentencing Reform Act, a bill that created United States Sentencing Commission, which was charged with creating minimum sentences for drug offenders convicted in federal court. Two years later, Congress passed the Anti-Drug Abuse Act, which required mandatory minimum sentences for the possession of narcotics. A defendant caught with five grams of crack cocaine (one or two very small rocks), for example, would be given a mandatory sentence of between 5 and 40 years in prison without probation or parole.

The Anti-Drug Abuse Act required a minimum of 10 years to life for a first drug conviction, 20 years to life for a second, and life in prison if the possession could be tied to a death or serious bodily injury.[27] These sentences applied to illegal drugs such as heroin, cocaine, and marijuana, as well as to legal drugs sold on the black market—pain relievers and sedatives, for example.

One consequence of mandatory drug sentencing is that sentencing power has been transferred from judges to prosecutors (and legislatures). Prosecutors now have the power to determine whether a case will be prosecuted in federal or state court. In many cases, they also have the option of selecting among several states, inevitably selecting the one that offers the harshest sentencing laws. This gives prosecutors enormous coercive power to pressure anyone accused of a drug offense to plead guilty in return for a lesser penalty.[28] It also leads to first-time drug offenders being sentenced as hardened criminals.

The Reagan administration also sponsored the Comprehensive Crime Control Act of 1984, which empowered the Department of Justice (DOJ) to seize assets derived from drug trafficking.[29] The legislation required the Justice Department to share seized assets with state and local law enforcement agencies assisting with the investigations. The assets of suspected drug offenders are seized without hearings or trial and thus are stripped of the resources they need to hire attorneys to defend themselves. Most are forced to rely upon inexperienced public defenders.[30]

In the aftermath of September 11, 2001, the Bush administration gave renewed impetus to the war on drugs by associating drug trafficking with terrorism. In 2002, for example, Attorney General John Ashcroft declared that "terrorism and drugs go together like rats and the bubonic plague."[31] He said that there is an "evil interdependence" between terrorists who kill Americans, and illegal drugs that make citizens slaves of drug addition. Ashcroft and the White House Office of National Drug Control Policy (ONDCP) have pointed out that nearly half of the terrorist organizations listed by the State Department had links to drug activity. ONDCP began running commercials during the 2002 Super Bowl establishing the link between drug use and international terrorism. On the accompanying Web site, ONDCP noted that the Taliban collected revenue from opium and heroin smuggling, for example, and that Columbian terrorists funded themselves through the narcotics trade. Terrorists are drug traffickers, the government said, and they finance themselves by addicting Americans.

The federal government advertisement of a link between terrorism and drug use doesn't stop with illicit drugs. Physicians who prescribe large amounts of pain-relieving narcotics to addicts have been swept up in the war on terror, too. Just before Dr. William Hurwitz, a highly respected pain doctor, was arrested in September 2003, Assistant U.S. Attorney Gene Rossi told the *Washington Post,* "our office will try our best to root out (prescription pain doctors) like the Taliban," a quote that either links doctors to terrorists, or reveals an indiscriminate, war-like mentality among federal prosecutors.[32]

Mandatory drug sentences have resulted in a dramatic increase in the prison population of the country. In 1970, drug offenders represented just 3,384 or 16.3 percent of the 20,686 federal prisoners. In 2002, that number jumped to about 70,000, or 54.7 percent of the 128,090 federal prisoners.[33] Between 1990 and 1995 alone, the number of drug-related arrests jumped 27 percent. In 1994, the DOJ reported that 21.5 percent of federal prisoners were "low-level offenders with no record of violence, involvement in sophisticated criminal activity, and no prior prison record."[34]

HISTORICAL PARALLELS IN THE WAR ON DOCTORS

There are several historical parallels between the contemporary war on doctors in the United States and the early-twentieth-century prosecutions under the Harrison Act. From 1915 until the end of Prohibition in 1933, thousands of innocent physicians were prosecuted as drug dealers under the Act, which drew heavy support from the temperance movement. With the endorsement of powerful mouthpieces such as Secretary of State William Jennings Bryan, Captain Richmond Pearson Hobson, the "Great Destroyer" of alcohol and narcotics addiction and the Anti-Saloon League's highest paid publicist, and Harry J. Anslinger, the first Commissioner of Narcotics and former Assistant Commissioner of Prohibition, the government inaugurated a reign of terror against physicians and their addicted patients. Because addicts were a small minority of the population and were largely powerless, they were the perfect target for eager prosecutors with political ambition. Politicians who wished to be seen as tough on law and order invariably focused their attention upon the alleged criminal behavior of these doctors and their drug addicts.

The Harrison Narcotics Act was repealed in 1970, but its legacy lives on. It was quickly replaced by the Drug Abuse Prevention and Control Act (DAPCA).[35] DAPCA, along with the 1975 Supreme Court ruling in the case *U.S. v. Moore*, reaffirmed the Harrison Act's criminalization of doctors who treat addicts by prescribing controlled pharmaceuticals.[36] In *United States v. Moore*, the Supreme Court confirmed that physicians who are licensed by the DEA to prescribe narcotics under Title II of the DAPCA (called the federal Controlled Substances Act (CSA) "can be prosecuted when their activities fall outside the usual course of professional practice."[37] A doctor could be criminally charged with unlawfully prescribing (or "diverting") highly addictive narcotic drugs that the DEA classifies as Schedule II "Controlled Substances."

The DEA Reverts to Its Original Mission

As the federal government's chief drug law enforcement agency since 1973, the DEA's mission is to "bring to the criminal and civil justice system substances destined for illicit traffic in the U.S."[38] Until the 1990s, the DEA focused its mission primarily upon illegal black market drugs such as heroin, cocaine, "crack" cocaine, ecstasy, and marijuana in urban areas of the country.

But in 1999, the DEA came under heavy criticism from Congress on the grounds that there was no "measurable proof" that it had reduced the illegal drug supply in the country.[39] In 2000 and 2001 the DOJ, which administrates the DEA, gave the agency a highly critical rebuke, and asserted that the DEA's goals were not consistent with the president's federal National Drug Control Strategy.[40] The DEA would need to find a new front for the war on drugs, one that could produce tangible, measurable results. Pain doctors were an available target.

Title II of the Drug Abuse Prevention and Control Act of 1970, called the Controlled Substances Act (CSA), empowered the DEA to regulate all pharmaceutical drugs. In 2002, Glen A. Fine, the Inspector General of the DOJ, asked why the DEA wasn't doing more to combat prescription drug abuse when it was a "problem equal to cocaine."[41] Fine claimed that 4.1 million Americans used cocaine in 2001, while 6.4 million illegally used narcotic painkillers the same year. He also claimed that the illicit use of pain medication accounted for 30 percent of all emergency room drug-related deaths and injuries. The DEA responded. The agency underscored the threat of prescription drug abuse by asserting that the number of people who "abuse controlled pharmaceuticals each year equals the number who abuse cocaine—2 to 4 percent of the U.S. population." The agency also claimed that prescription drugs increased the number of overdose deaths by 25 percent and accounted for 20 percent of all emergency room visits for drug overdoses.

The DEA responded to its congressional critics by announcing a major new antidrug campaign, the OxyContin Action Plan.[42] The plan elevated a legal, prescription drug to a status equivalent to the most dangerous illegal drug in the country-cocaine. Since only physicians can prescribe narcotics, the DEA's policy shift has made doctors targets for investigation as illegal drug dealers. This explains, for example, assistant U.S. Attorney Mark Lytle's claim in September 2003, at Dr. Hurwitz's 69-count indictment, that he was guilty of distributing dangerous drugs on the black market leading to the deaths of three patients. Lytle compared William Hurwitz to a "street-corner crack dealer" and said that he should not be treated any differently from a crack dealer because he had a medical degree. Indeed, Lytle said that Dr. Hurwitz was so dangerous to the community that he should be denied bail.[43]

In many ways, the OxyContin Action Plan resembled the Harrison Act—it outlawed a previously legal narcotic drug due to unfounded fears of a "dope menace" sweeping the country. DEA Commissioner Asa Hutchinson said the nonmedical use of OxyContin constituted a deadly new drug epidemic spreading throughout towns and cities in the rural heartland of America. He said that the epidemic began in Appalachia and was a growing problem spreading from the Eastern States to suburban and urban areas throughout the nation. Hutchinson said:

> In the past, Americans viewed drug abuse and addiction as an overwhelmingly urban problem. As the drug problem escalated, drugs began to stream into rural neighborhoods throughout small town America. Residents began to feel the impact of drugs such as marijuana, cocaine, methamphetamine, MDMA, heroin, and *OxyContin* which entered their towns at an alarming rate. Violence associated with drug trafficking also became part of the landscape in small cities and rural areas.[44]

This was the first time that the DEA had classified a legal, prescription drug with dangerous, illegal drugs such as cocaine and heroin. During congressional testimony in April 2002, Hutchinson explained the necessity for renewed vigilance in the war on drugs, and why opening this new front against prescription painkillers was necessary. Hutchinson declared that the DEA would reallocate its resources from illegal drugs in urban areas to illicit prescription drugs in rural areas in order to balance this emerging drug threat. To this end, he said that the DEA work with local and state law enforcement agencies and would use its Asset Forfeiture Fund to augment the meager resources of state and local agencies to deal with this new drug problem.[45]

The DEA's association of the highly popular pain relief drug OxyContin with illegal drugs was a marked departure from the conventional war on drugs. Instead of banning or eliminating OxyContin, the DEA declared that the legal drug was a public menace, comparable to that of cocaine and heroin. Consequently, the DEA created a new mission for itself—combating the illegal diversion of otherwise legal medication.

Justifying the OxyContin Campaign

In an effort to justify its national campaign against OxyContin, the DEA contacted 775 medical examiners from the National Association of Medical Examiners in 2001 and instructed them to report "OxyContin-related deaths" in 2000 and 2001.[46] Based upon these autopsy reports, the DEA claimed that there were 464 OxyContin-related deaths in those two years.[47]

But the DEA's report contains some notable flaws. First, there is no test to distinguish OxyContin from any of the other 58 drug products that also contain oxycodone (the active narcotic agent in OxyContin).[48] OxyContin is merely the Purdue Pharma brand name for one of three single entity oxycodone pain medications that are long-acting and high-dosage (making them ideal for chronic pain sufferers). Other brand name oxycodone products—Percocet, Percodan, and Roxicet, for example—have a lower dosage, are short-acting, and are supplemented by nonnarcotic pain relievers such as aspirin and Tylenol.

Second, the DEA's criterion for what it calls "OxyContin-related deaths" is also problematic. According to the agency, if oxycodone is detected by a medical examiner in an autopsy without the presence of aspirin or Tylenol, the deceased is automatically counted as an "OxyContin-likely death." If an OxyContin tablet is found in the gastrointestinal tract of a deceased, the deceased is labeled an "OxyContin-verified death." Likewise, if investigators find OxyContin pills or prescriptions at a crime scene, or a family member or witness reports the presence of OxyContin, the death is again confirmed as "OxyContin-verified." Obviously the mere presence of OxyContin in the system of the deceased or the mere mention of the drug by friends or family members is far from verification that OxyContin—either alone or in conjunction with other factors—actually caused the death. But for DEA public relations purposes, it's close enough.

Another problem with the DEA's definition of an OxyContin death is that most overdose victims have multiple drugs in their bodies. Approximately 40 percent of the autopsy reports of OxyContin-related deaths showed the presence of Valium-like drugs. Another 40 percent contained an additional opiate such as Percodan, Vicodan, Lortab, or Lorcet in addition to oxycodone. Thirty percent showed an antidepressant such as Prozac, 15 percent showed cocaine, and 14 percent indicated the presence of over-the-counter antihistamines or cold medications. Deaths like these cannot reliably be attributed to any particular drug. They could be the result of any of the drugs present, drugs working in combination, or one or more drugs plus the effects of other conditions, such as illness or disease. Indeed, the March 2003 issue of the *Journal of Analytical Toxicology* found that of the 919 deaths related to oxycodone in 23 states over a three-year period, only 12 showed confirmed evidence that presence of OxyContin alone in the system of the deceased.[49] About 70 percent of the deaths were due to "multiple drug poisoning" of other oxycodone-containing drugs in combination with Valium-type tranquilizers, alcohol, cocaine, marijuana, other narcotics, and antidepressants. This is pretty strong evidence that many of the deaths attributable to OxyContin are not the result of unknowing pain patients who grew addicted and overdosed, but of habitual drug users who may have used the drug with any number of other substances, any one of which could have contributed to death.

A final problem with the DEA's claims of an OxyContin epidemic is the agency's overly cautious estimate of risk of death. In 2000, there were 7.1 million prescriptions of oxycodone products without aspirin or Tylenol, 5.8 million of them OxyContin.[50] According to the DEA's own autopsy data, there were 146 "OxyContin-verified deaths" that year, and 318 "OxyContin-likely deaths." That makes for a total of 464 "OxyContin-related deaths."[51] That amounts to a risk of just 0.00008 percent, or 8 deaths per 100,000 OxyContin prescriptions—2.5 "verified" and 5.5 "likely related." And that's only after taking the DEA's troubling conclusions about causation at face value. Given these numbers, it's quite a stretch to claim that OxyContin abuse amounts to a deadly drug epidemic sweeping the heartland of America.

A New Drug Hysteria

In order for the DEA to justify its new mission in the war on drugs, the government had to persuade the public that there was a major new drug threat facing the country. Given the country's long history of demonizing drug addicts and dealers as the source of crime and misery, it was relatively easy to bring the media along, and ultimately generate public support for the DEA's latest mission.[52]

Since the 1980s, the government has reported that cocaine, especially in its crack form, is the "principal drug threat to the United States."[53] The National Drug Threat Survey (NDTS) data showed that 33.1 percent of state and local law enforcement agencies regard cocaine (powder and crack) as the greatest drug threat to the country. Shortly after the DEA announced its renewed war on drugs in the mid-1980s, the media followed with an explosion of reports linking drug-related violence to crack cocaine. In 1986, for example, *Newsweek* reported that crack "spawns vicious violence among dealers and dopers creating an epidemic of urban lawlessness."[54]

To set the stage for the opioid drug threat, the DEA would need to compare OxyContin to crack, cocaine, and heroin, chief demon drugs of the 1980s and

1990s. And it did. For example, Asa Hutchinson testified before Congress in 2002 that OxyContin delivers a "heroin-like high" and that the drug has led to an "increase in criminal activity."[55] The fits a familiar pattern in the government's war on drugs. Drug use equals abuse that constitutes a problem leading to a national drug crisis. Over the last few years, taking their cues from the DEA, hundreds of newspapers and magazines have sensationalized the threat of this new killer drug sweeping the country.

Beginning in 2000 the media has portrayed OxyContin as a highly addictive, dangerous, and potent narcotic with a "heroin-like" high. The media jumped on an alleged rising death toll from OxyContin, and that the outbreak in opioid abuse posed a threat greater threat to public health and welfare than cocaine. With a few quotes about death statistics, arrests, and company sales of OxyContin, the media had thus helped the DEA to fabricate a new drug threat, one in which an American pharmaceutical company was allegedly fueling addiction and death across the country.

A few examples of media stories describing the threat that OxyContin poses are given below.

On May 21, 2000, the *Boston Globe* ran a story quoting a local sheriff, Joseph Tibbetts, in Maine who said that the inmate population of his 40-bed jail was filled with people caught committing armed robberies in search of a "heroin-like narcotics"—OxyContin.[56] The jail was full of people convicted of break-ins and armed robberies to get cash to pay for OxyContin they can obtain from doctors' prescriptions. Tibbetts described OxyContin use in remote Washington County with a population of 36,000, as "a social epidemic" and said that no "home is unaffected" by it.

On January 8, 2001, Time Magazine ran a story reporting that "OxyContin may succeed crack cocaine on the street."[57] The story claimed that OxyContin was becoming a dangerous drug throughout the country. The police in the New Orleans suburb of St. Bernard Parish described OxyContin abuse as an "epidemic" and they were making many arrests for the "killers" who were selling the drug. The author said that OxyContin was so popular and addictive that it had "stirred up a blizzard of a crime wave." In Pulaska, Virigina, Oxy-Contin had overtaken cocaine and marijuana and property crime was up 50 percent according to the police chief.

The police in three states reported a record number of pharmacies robberies and the homes of people with legitimate OxyContin prescriptions were being invaded to obtain the drug. According to U.S. Attorney Jay McCloskey who was "waging a war against the doctors who write prescriptions," Maine is the second largest consumer of OxyContin and it had 35 deaths from overdoses in 2000.

On February 3, 2001, US News & World Report published an article about the danger of OxyContin entitled "The Poor Man's Heroin."[58] The article features Dr. John F. Lilly, a 48-year-old orthopedist who opened a pain clinic. Prosecutors claimed that Dr. Lilly was running a "pill mill" that supplied illegal narcotics to addicts in the slums of the industrial city of Portsmouth, Ohio.

Local law enforcement officials reported that OxyContin abuse was reaching near-epidemic levels in rural areas. Shortly after Dr. Lilly opened his clinic, drug-related crimes started to rise. The police claimed that burglaries increased 20 percent over 2000. According to a pharmacologist with Ohio Drug and Poison Control, "when people become aware of a script doctor they come in droves." He elaborated that "drug abuse goes through fads and epidemics and OxyContin is on the upturn."

On February 8, 2001, the *New York Times* reported a claim by U.S. attorney Joseph Famularo that at least 59 people had died from OxyContin overdoses in eastern Kentucky in 2000.[59] He claimed that OxyContin has set off a wave of pharmacy burglaries, emergency room visits and arrests of doctors. The problem was so urgent in Kentucky that on February 6, 2001, more than 100 Kentucky police joined in drug raids over a five-county area netting 207 suspects in one week during Operation Oxyfest 2001.

Captain Minor Allen of the Hazard Police Department in Kentucky described the situation in southeastern Kentucky as an epidemic. He said that there was a "growing drug culture" of high-school students and young people in the twenties in "Pillville." The "new addiction" was a rootless population that was not previously involved in drug trafficking. Roy W. Hatfield, the police chief of Harlan, Kentucky, said that OxyContin was "pushing out" marijuana and barbiturates. Rick Moorer, an investigator with the state medical examiner's office in Roanoke, Virginia, reported that there were 16 deaths in southwestern Virginia due to OxyContin in combination with other drugs and alcohol.

The article used federation data showing hospital emergency room visits by people on oxycodone increased from 3,190 in 1996 to 6,429 in 1999. This purportedly reflected the impact of OxyContin that was released in 1996. They quoted a bulletin by the National Drug Intelligence Center warning that misuse of OxyContin was concentrated in the East but was spreading throughout the country.

One of the more egregious examples of media-induced OxyContin hysteria was Doris Bloodsworth's five-part *Orlando Sentinel* series from October 19–23, 2003, entitled "OxyContin Under Fire."[60] Bloodsworth, described herself as a "mom with a word processor who always wanted to be a reporter." She spread the OxyContin drug hysteria, sponsored by the DEA, with alacrity in order to advance her career. She began researching the effects of OxyContin in December 2002, shortly after attending a drug convention.[61]

The series was designed to expose a deadly OxyContin epidemic sweeping the country. It included 19 articles replete with photos of victims, flashy layouts, and insert boxes designed for maximum emotional impact upon readers. The series featured patients who supposedly were accidentally addicted to OxyContin. Some of them experienced painful withdrawal and detoxification, accidental overdose deaths, suicide, and the destruction of their families. She claimed that the most likely people to die from this epidemic were white males from ages 30 to 60, with back pain.[62]

The series featured David Rokisky, a 36-year-old former Army Airborne soldier and police officer living in Tampa, Florida. According to Bloodsworth, Rokisky had a bodybuilder's physique, a beautiful young wife, a high-paying job as a computer-company executive, and a beach-front condo. He had an idyllic life until a doctor prescribed OxyContin to treat a minor backache and he became an innocent victim of drug addiction, lost his job, and had to undergo detoxification. The series also featured Gerry Cover, a 39-year-old Kissimmee, Florida, handyman and father of three, who became an addict after a doctor prescribed OxyContin to relieve his pain from a mild herniated disc in his back. Cover subsequently died from an accidental overdose of the drug.

Bloodsworth said that while members of Congress and the FDA were aware of the devastation (OxyContin) has carved through Appalachia where the drug became known as "hillbilly heroin," nothing was being done to stop the deadly drug epidemic. She blamed the drug's manufacturer, Purdue Pharma, for aggressively marketing OxyContin to naïve and unscrupulous doctors who used the drug to "boost their profits."

The unregulated distribution of OxyContin was producing death and destruction in its wake. According to Bloodsworth, from 2001 to 2002, there were 573 deaths in Florida linked to oxycodone (the active ingredient in OxyContin). This was based upon the paper's painstaking review of thousands of documents including 500 autopsy reports by Florida's Medical Examiners for those years. The paper claimed that 83 percent of the 247 cases of reported drug overdose deaths were attributed to OxyContin. By comparison, Bloodsworth said that only "521 people died of heroin overdoses during the same period." The *Sentinel* also claimed to have studied the personal health histories 303 of the 500 overdose victims studied. They found that 87 patients had suffered from back pain or injuries while only 38 overdose deaths were due to drug abuse.

The series contributed to the national OxyContin drug hysteria. It not only started a grassroots protest movement in Florida but it prompted state and federal politicians to take action to deal with the new drug epidemic. In November 2003, one month after the series appeared, protestors from all over the country converged in Florida to picket Governor Jeb Bush and his wife who were attending a three-day conference on youth drug abuse in Orlando. They called themselves Relatives Against Purdue Pharma and carried poster-sized photos of family members and friends who allegedly died from OxyContin overdoses.[63] For example, Victor Del Regno, a Rhode Island business executive whose 20-year-old son died from OxyContin said, "We feel there has to be a way to get the word out about how deadly this drug can be."[64]

The governor and state politicians took up the cause and promised to put an end to the deadly prescription drug epidemic and stop the "hemorrhaging of lost lives."[65] During congressional testimony, James McDonough, the governor's director of drug control cited Doris Bloodsworth's series including her estimates of OxyContin overdose deaths. He said that in response to the *Sentinel* and other reports, Florida had taken "aggressive action against criminal practices" including the conviction of Dr. James Graves for four counts of manslaughter for prescribing oxycodone, Dr. Sarfraz Mirza for trafficking in OxyContin, and Dr. Michell Wich and Dr. Asuncion Luyao for prescription overdose deaths.[66]

Bloodsworth's claims about the OxyContin epidemic was picked up and repeated in newspaper and media throughout the country. It was even included in a GAO government report on OxyContin abuse requested by Congress. The study cited the *Sentinel* series and said that the newspaper's investigation of autopsy reports involving oxycodone-related deaths found that "OxyContin had been involved in over 200 overdose deaths in Florida since 2000."[67]

The *Sentinel* Series Unravels

In February 2004, the *Orlando Sentinel* series began to fall apart. Investigations by Purdue Pharma and advocates of pain patients who depend upon opiates to live normal lives uncovered numerous errors in the reports. On February 16, the *Washington Post* reported, for example, that David Rokisky, the lead character in the series had, in fact, pleaded guilty to a federal drug conspiracy in a cocaine case four years before the series appeared. Far from having an idyllic life until taking OxyContin, Rokisky had a long history of domestic-abuse allegations and financial problems.[68] In an effort to demonize OxyContin, Rokisky and others in the series were misrepresented as "accidental" victims of addiction. Another so-called innocent victim of prescription addiction, Gerry Cover, was actually a drug addict and had overdosed on other drugs three months before being prescribed OxyContin.[69]

The series' misrepresentation of OxyContin overdose deaths was even more egregious than the mischaracterization of the alleged victims of the drug. The series completely distorted the Florida Medical Examiners' reports of drug overdose deaths for years 2000 and 2001. Instead of more than 200 deaths linked to OxyContin, the medical examiners' reports reveals the actual total for those years was 71—35 in 2001, and 36 in 2002.[70] The *Sentinel* had included not only oxycodone-only related deaths, but also deaths where oxycodone was present in combination with any number of other drugs. There were 317 such deaths in 2001 and 220 in 2002, giving the *Sentinel* its 573 deaths. In truth, even those 71 overdose deaths over the *Sentinel's* two-year period were questionable. That is because Florida's medical examiners report only 14 drug groups in their autopsy reports.[71] It is likely that there were other nonreported drugs in the systems of the deceased, not to mention possible causes of death unrelated to drugs. For example, the deceased may also have been taking antidepressants, heart medication, and/or diabetic medications, any of which could have potentially contributed to the cause of death. That is particularly likely where the deceased were over 50 years of age—true of about a third of the cases.[72]

After receiving a barrage of criticism for three months, the *Orlando Sentinel* finally acknowledged errors in the series and in February 2004, they announced Doris Bloodsworth's resignation from the paper and the reassignment of two editors who worked on the series.[73] Despite the embarrassment to the newspaper, the fear of an OxyContin epidemic sweeping the country has continued in Florida and elsewhere in the country. For example, on March 3, 2004, the *Sun-Sentinel* in Ft. Lauderdale, Florida, a sister paper to the *Orlando Sentinel*, both owned by the *Chicago Tribune*, published a story about the arrest of a doctor in Jupiter, Florida, Dr. Denis Deonarine who was charged with first-degree murder for the overdose death of a patient whom he had prescribed OxyContin.[74] In October 2004, Marc Kaufman writing for the *Washington Post*, repeated the OxyContin epidemic fear when he reported that "OxyContin became popular with drug abusers especially in rural and southern areas, and it has been linked to numerous hospitalizations and some deaths."[75] He noted that scores of pain doctors have been convicted of drug offenses and have been sent to prison for decades.

Eradicating the Prescription Painkiller "Threat"

Given the large number of pain patients and doctors who treat them, the DEA's new mission to thwart the "diversion" of prescription painkillers would be a huge undertaking, one that would require significant manpower and resources. From May 2001, the initiation of the OxyContin Action Plan, to January 2004, the DEA carried out over 400 investigations resulting in the arrest of 600 individuals. Sixty percent of the cases were medical professionals such as doctors and pharmacists.[76]

In order to carry out this new program, the DEA participates in the Organized Crime Drug Enforcement Task Force (OCDETF) and works cooperatively with state and local drug task forces. This combines the resources of federal, state, and local law enforcement under the coordination of the U.S. attorneys. In 2001, the DEA deputized 1,554 state and local officers from large and small police departments across the country to coordinate drug investigations. In 2002, there were 1,172 DEA special agents working alongside 1,916 state and local police officers in 207 separate task forces.[77]

In 1999, for example, the DEA initiated 1,699 cases on its own but amplified its investigative reach by working cooperatively with state and local law enforcement officials in more than 9,000 task force cases.[78] The DEA also trained more than 64,000 state and local law enforcement personnel in 2001 at its Training Academy in Quantico, Virginia, and at the agency's 22 domestic field divisions throughout the United States.[79] These task forces accounted for 40 percent of the DEA's prescription narcotics seizure and forfeiture cases.[80]

The DEA's Diversion Control Program is also a self-financing, autonomous law enforcement agency that is largely unaccountable. It's mostly financed by the licenses it requires all doctors, manufacturers, pharmacists, and wholesalers to purchase, and in part by what the assets it seizes when it raids the businesses and personal finances of those same licensees.Table 7.1 shows the

Table 7.1
DEA Registrant Population

Retail Level		Wholesale Level	
Practitioner (doctors)	928,677	Researchers	6,843
Nurse practitioners & physicians' assistants	71,169	Analytical labs	1,591
Pharmacies	61,057	Narcotic programs	1,151
Hospitals/clinics	14,462	Distributors	876
Teaching institutions	424	Manufacturers	453
Importers	136	Exporters	206

Source: DEA Update, National Association of State Controlled Substance Authorities, Myrtle Beach, South Carolina, October 2002.

breakdown of the DEA's controlled substance license holders as of 2002. Physicians constituted 928,677 of 1,087,045 registrants, or 85 percent of all those approved by the DEA to produce, distribute, and dispense narcotics. Because prescription narcotics are legal, the DEA is able to monitor the way physicians prescribe them. Unlike illicit drug dealers, physicians are legal, legitimate professionals. They behave rationally. That also makes them easier targets for the DEA.

The DEA also sets annual production quotas for the manufacturers of narcotic drugs, and the agency attempts to monitor the wholesale and retail distribution of those drugs, though with decidedly mixed results. In fact, large quantities of narcotics routinely go missing en route from manufacturers, to wholesalers, to retailers. The DEA itself acknowledges the problem. They note that there is an increase in OxyContin burglaries, thefts, and robberies of hospitals and pharmacies throughout the country including Purdue Pharma, the manufacturer of OxyContin.[81]

In one recent case in Arizona, nearly 475,000 tablets of narcotic drugs disappeared from Kino Community Hospital's pharmacy between May 1, 2002 to April 30, 2004.[82] Drug Stores in rural areas have been targets for burglars seeking OxyContin and the Internet has become a major source for the drug.[83] *The Star-Ledger* newspaper in New Jersey went so far as to successfully order OxyContin along with other narcotics over the Internet. There was no contact with a physician and the drugs were delivered to a rented mailbox within days of placing the order.[84]

In 1993, Congress created the self-financed Diversion Control Fund, which was to be funded by narcotics licensing fees. The DEA is obligated to increase the license fees to make sure the Diversion Control Program (DCP) remains fully funded. The setup is similar to that of the Health Care Fraud and Abuse Control Program (HCFACP), which monitors doctors for alleged fraud and abuse. In 2003, the DEA doubled its license fees in order to pay for the cost of the program. Under DEA rules, doctors must buy licenses for three year periods at $131 per annum per physician, and $1,605 per annum for pharmaceutical companies to make drugs. These licensing fees bring in about $118 million a year. The DCP currently costs about $154 million per year.

The rest of the funding comes from the annual congressional budget for the DEA and from the DOJ's Asset Forfeiture Fund, which is financed by seizures of assets from doctors and pharmacists under investigation for drug diversion plus illegal drug dealers and users. According to the CSA, all moneys or other things of value furnished by any person in exchange for controlled substances are subject to forfeiture.[85]

This diversion forfeiture money is deposited in the DOJ's Forfeiture Fund that is used to coordinate investigations and prosecutions of physicians and pharmacists with state and local law enforcement agencies. In 2002, drug asset forfeitures were $441 million. And in 2001, the DEA shared $179,264,498 of its asset forfeitures with local and state police departments.[86] The Attorney General controls the forfeiture fund that was worth more than $1.2 billion in 2002.[87] Through an asset-sharing program, the vast majority of asset forfeiture money is distributed by the DEA to state and local law enforcement agencies who work with the agency on cases. It is a perverse system that in essence allows cops to keep for their departments the assets of suspected drug defendants.

Detective Dennis M. Luken of the Warren-Clinton Drug & Strategic Operations Task Force in Lebanon, Ohio, and the Treasurer of the National Association of Diversion Drug Investigators (NADDI), explained the financial importance of targeting physicians for investigation.[88] Luken, who worked on an asset forfeiture squad for three and a half years, said that in an "era of budget cuts, forfeitures are an important way to make up for the losses."[89] Luken said that the task force arrests five doctors a year in the Cincinnati area alone. John Burke, the vice president of NADDI, and Luken's commander in Ohio, and a consultant to Purdue Pharma, the manufacturer of OxyContin, said that "prescription drugs are as addictive as the vast majority of street drugs and (one percent or about 10,000) physicians cause hundreds of thousands of addicts and are nothing less than drug dealers, regardless of the license or shingle they hang at their office."[90]

Seizing doctor's assets was a recurring theme at a NAAI training conference held in Ft. Lauderdale, Florida, in July 2003. For example, Greg Aspinwall of the Miami Dade Drug Task Force stressed the importance of taking a task force approach to diversion investigations by using the theme "spreading the love."[91] He said that as many law enforcement agencies as possible should be involved in investigations; it reduces the cost and guarantees that "everybody gets their fair cut from the forfeitures."[92] He noted that even if there were no criminal charges, they can bring civil action to recover the cost of an investigation.

RECENT FORFEITURES ENUMERATED BY THE OHIO TASK FORCE

Luken focused upon "drug diverting" doctors and stressed the importance of seizing their assets. He urged investigators to serve search warrants on doctors' office and bank accounts and seizing their funds. If the doctor does not have a sizable bank account, they should seize their office buildings since it was paid for from the proceeds of dealing drugs. Luken implored agents to "remember that asset forfeiture investigation should begin at the start of your criminal case."[93] It is instructive to list a few of the physicians that Detective Luken discussed in light of the property and money that investigators seized from them *before* they were indicted or tried for any crime.

- Dr. Joseph Massoud was investigated for billing for visiting multiple nursing homes. He surrendered his medical license and DEA license and the task force seized $9,000 from him as forfeited funds.
- Dr. John Lyons was investigated for billing fraud and deception to obtain dangerous drugs. He surrendered his medical license, DEA license and they seized $12,174 from his bank account and demanded $30,000 more to avoid taking his office building.
- Dr. Glenn Heigerick, 75-year-old doctor, was investigated for billing fraud and selling the drug, phentermine from his office. He surrendered his medical and DEA licenses and was ordered to pay $100,000 in asset forfeiture (cash and office building).
- Dr. Eli Schneider was investigated for billing fraud and illegally prescribing dangerous drugs. His bank account was frozen and the task force seized $220,000. The money was distributed in the following amounts. The Ohio Medicaid Fraud Control Unit received $3,752.04, the Ohio Department of Human Services got $24,000, the Cincinnati Police Department received $29,000, the FBI got $14,000, and the U.S. Department of Health and Human Services collected $50,000. Dr. Schneider ultimately only had $100,000 of his money returned to him.

As the DCP is self-financed, it is not under the control of Congress. It does not need to justify its existence or its efficacy when it comes time for appropriations. It also creates a Kafkaesque scenario where doctors are required to finance potential investigations of their practices, which could lead to the seizure of everything they own, which then goes toward financing more investigations.

From October 1999 through March 2002, the DEA investigated 247 OxyContin diversion cases leading to 328 arrests.[94] In 2001, there were 3,097 total (including OxyContin) diversion investigations, including 861 investigations of doctors.[95] In 2003, the DEA investigated 732 doctors, sanctioned 584, and arrested 50.[96]

These numbers include just the DEA cases. They do not include physicians investigated and arrested by the 217 DEA state and local task forces throughout the country.

Misplaced Tactics

The DEA defines addicts as individuals who habitually use any narcotic drug that endangers the public morals, health, safety, or welfare.[97] The DEA includes in that definition the millions of patients who depend upon narcotics for pain relief. Chronic noncancerous pain patients who are prescribed large amounts of narcotics, then, are addicts—or, given draconian drug laws that say possession of any controlled substance over a specified amount is de facto intent to distribute, they are often "dealers," too. That also means that the doctors who treat these patients are conspirators in the illegal drug trade.

Narcotics investigators focus upon physicians, pharmacists, and dentists as major sources of drug diversion.[98] According to Detective Luken, like illegal drug dealers, doctors sell drugs for money, sex, or to feed their drug habits or those of family members or girlfriends. Doctors who are in practice by themselves and older doctors were also said to be prone to illegally divert drugs because they are easily duped or continue to prescribe narcotics as they had during a more permissive era.[99]

In order to target drug-dealing doctors, investigators look for "red flags" they believe are indicative of potentially criminal behavior. These red flags are circumstantial evidence based on standard criminal investigative procedures. The problem with red flags is that what may appear to be evidence of criminal behavior to a medically naïve investigator is often a characteristic of legitimate medical practice. Criminal investigators without medical training simply are not qualified to tell the difference.

Prosecutions of doctors are based on whether there is "legitimate medical purpose" for a drug prescription or whether it is "beyond the bounds of medical practice." But prosecutors concede that there are no specific guidelines to prove a doctor's actions are without a legitimate medical purpose, or that they acted outside the bounds of their professional medical practice. According to a federal investigator who addressed a Healthcare Fraud Prevention & Funds Recovery Summit in Washington, DC, in 2004, the government seeks to produce probable cause that a doctor intentionally wrote a narcotics prescription for patients without legitimate medical needs or knew the patients were addicts or were selling the drugs.[100]

An illustration of the controversial nature of red flags as the basis for investigating and prosecuting physicians was the DEA's rejection of a "Frequently Asked Questions (FAQ)" document in November 2004. The FAQ was the combined product of leading physicians and researchers in pain medicine and the DEA working collaboratively from 2001.[101] The purpose of the document was to provide a guideline for doctors who prescribe narcotics to pain patients, and law enforcement agents who investigate doctors for drug diversion. The DEA took the extraordinary step of disavowing the document shortly after they posted it on their own Web site. The agency issued an interim statement disavowing the FAQ. The reason the DEA gave for rejecting the document was that it contained errors.

The errors turned out to be the DEA's insistence that they are not bound by any "standard of evidentiary requirement to commence an investigation" including the well-established principal in federal law that the enforcement of the CSA should in no way interfere the ethical practice of medicine.[102] In other words, the DEA would continue to use red flags of criminality when deciding to investigate doctors. The red flags specifically in the interim policy statement included the number of tablets a doctor prescribed to his patients, writing more than one prescription for a patient on the same day and marked for later dispensing, and using "street slang" rather than medical terminology.

This means that investigators and prosecutors without medical training must interpret physicians' actions in order to get criminal convictions. Thus, the need for red flags. The NADDI instructs cops to conduct video surveillance of doctors' offices as if they were "crack houses."[103] At the July 2003 NADDI conference, investigators were told what practices—red flags—might indicate criminal behavior. They include:

- Long lines of patients waiting to see doctors.
- Patients who are poorly dressed.
- Out-of-state automobile licenses in doctors' parking lots.
- Patients who arrive and are taken without appointments.
- Patient visits lasting less than 25 minutes.
- Doctors who are licensed to practice in more than one state.
- Doctors who dispense large amounts of narcotics from one office.

Investigators also picked through trash at doctors' offices and at their homes, looking for incriminating evidence. Employees of suspected doctors were interviewed at their homes, and police searched for disgruntled former employees who would incriminate the doctors. Investigators sent undercover agents, typically from sheriffs' departments, to pose as pain patients with fake insurance cards. Agents scheduled appointments over the phone and carefully documented everything that happened during the office visits. They made audio and, when possible, video recordings of everything that occurred. Undercover agents tended to be females. Investigators believed women were less threatening, less suspicious, and more likely to illicit sympathy from doctors. Undercover agents made numerous visits within short intervals to doctor's offices in order to befriend the staff, and gain their trust. They also attempted to accumulate incriminating evidence against the doctors. They were instructed to engage in informal, personal conversation with their "target" and his employees. Once an undercover agent won the trust of a doctor and his staff, he was instructed to begin looking for more "red flags." These included:

- A doctor who told a pain patient where he can get his prescriptions filled.
- A physician asked his patients which drugs they prefer, or which dosage works best for them.
- Doctors who prescribed the same drug in the same dosage to many patients, including members of the same family.

A doctor's billing practices also triggered a red flag. Investigators contacted private insurance companies' fraud units, as well as those within Medicare and Medicaid. They obtained the billing histories of the doctors. If a physician used the same billing code and charged, for example, $100 for patient office visits, it was a potential red flag. Investigators also obtained the prescription purchase reports gathered by the DEA from the pharmaceutical companies to track a suspected physician's prescribing history.

Once they had enough evidence for a warrant, police are told to raid a doctor's office at lunchtime or at the end of the day. Their search warrants ordered the seizure of records, including patient files and billing. They were told to photocopy the records and return a copy the next business day. They were instructed to get as many law enforcement agencies involved in the investigation as possible, in order to augment the police resources needed to gather and share incriminating evidence. They were instructed to seize all of a doctor's assets, including bank accounts. In effect, doctors were treated the same as cocaine or heroin dealers.

Dr. William Hurwitz—the case previously discussed that prompted the "Taliban" comment from a federal prosecutor—was eventually charged with "conspiring to traffic drugs, drug trafficking resulting in death and serious injury, engaging in a criminal enterprise and health care fraud." He was arrested at his home by 20 armed agents in the presence of his 2 young daughters. His assets were seized, including his retirement account, and he was jailed without bond. According to the *Washington Post,* Assistant U.S. Attorney Mark Lytle said in court that Hurwitz is no better than a crack dealer, simply because he has a medical degree.

Prosecutors did not have to prove a doctor's malicious intent or desire to profit from narcotics diversion. It is not even necessary for the government to have expert medical testimony that a doctor's actions were illegitimate or outside the usual course of professional practice. Prosecutors were able to convict doctors even if they did not distribute drugs or their prescriptions are not actually filled.

The single most valuable police informants were pharmacists, because they sold the drugs that doctors prescribed to patients. Pharmacists were part of law enforcement, operating as police informants. For example, if out-of-town patients who were nervous and perspiring, dirty or disheveled turn up at a pharmacy with a doctor's prescription for narcotics, pharmacists would often call the police. They would report the presence of addicts or drug dealers without ever talking to the doctor who wrote the prescription. These calls invariably triggered criminal investigations of physicians.

8

THE WITCH HUNT FOR "DRUG-DEALING" DOCTORS: JAMES GRAVES, M.D., AND FRANK FISHER, M.D.

Dr. James Graves was a family doctor specializing in pain management in Pace, Florida, in 2002, when he was tried and convicted for racketeering, drug trafficking, and manslaughter. Dr. Graves received a sentence of more than 62 years in prison. The Graves trial set a national precedent for prosecutors throughout the country. He was the first doctor to be convicted of manslaughter for prescribing painkillers to patients who overdosed on drugs and died.

The prosecutor in the case, Florida Assistant State Attorney Russ Edgar, called Graves' manslaughter conviction a "barrier breaker." He said that prosecutors had never before charged a doctor with manslaughter for prescribing a painkiller to their patients. Indeed, Edgar reported that he initially considered a first-degree murder charge against Graves. He said that bringing such charges against a doctor would be an even bigger barrier-breaker, but manslaughter would have to come first.

Russ Edgar compared Dr. Graves to a street drug dealer. He said that Graves' practice was like a vending machine. Patients paid him $50 or $60, mostly in cash, punched the buttons that corresponded with their fake symptoms, and then pulled the lever for their narcotics.

Edgar asserted that Dr. Graves bore complete responsibility for his patients' overdose deaths. In fact, he accused Graves of deliberately addicting patients to narcotics and then supplying them with drugs for money. Edgar made the following comment after the trial:

> Doctors who too freely prescribe new, more powerful narcotics are a danger to patients. The script doctors then become potential killers.[1]

The conviction of Dr. Graves for manslaughter in February 2002 set off a panic within the medical community, especially among physicians who treat chronic pain patients. Their fears were fully justified. The Graves case immediately became a national model for prosecutors throughout the country, and Russ Edgar became a celebrity among prosecutors.

After the trial, Edgar went on a speaking tour around the country addressing dozens of prosecutors and investigators at both state and federal levels. He even produced a CD outlining his prosecution strategy against Dr. Graves and gave PowerPoint seminars at conferences. Dr. Theodore Parran, an addiction expert at the Case Western Reserve University medical school who testified against Dr. Graves at the trial, elaborated on the significance of the case:

> My impression is that prosecutors have generally felt unwilling to push the manslaughter side of this because of not really having a game plan on how to make a manslaughter charge stick. The Graves case gives them a roadmap.[2]

Edgar's prosecution model was immediately adopted by prosecutors around the country. Soon after Graves' conviction, for example, three other doctors were charged with manslaughter using Edgar's prosecution theory.

Criminal investigations and trials were launched against Dr. Denis Deonarine of West Palm Beach, Florida, Dr. Cecil Knox of Roanoke, Virginia, and Dr. Frank Fisher of Redding, California. Even in the case of Dr. Fisher who was completely exonerated of all charges, his practice and personal life were shattered by Edgar's "barrier-breaking" theory of prosecution.

A New Prosecution Theory

The Graves case was the first successful attempt by the state to apply the Racketeer Influenced and Corrupt Organizations Act (RICO) of 1970 to a medical doctor. Dr. Graves was prosecuted for being the leader of a criminal enterprise. He was said to be operating an elaborate racketeering conspiracy through the façade of a medical practice.

RICO was originally enacted by Congress to eradicate organized crime by attacking the sources of revenue of gambling or bookmaking syndicates. It was an aggressive law enforcement initiative that gave prosecutors a new weapon of unprecedented scope for an assault on the economic roots of organized crime.

Ironically, RICO did not even mention organized crime. Instead, it used the term "racketeering activity." This term has become a catch-all phrase that includes a wide variety of crimes, including sexual abuse, drug trafficking, murder, kidnapping, gambling, arson, robbery, extortion, money laundering, mail fraud, price-fixing, bribery, extortion, fraud, embezzlement, and obscene material. Because of its wide-reaching scope, it has the potential for prosecutorial abuse. Indeed, RICO has been used against legitimate businesses, political groups, and even churches. Almost anyone can be targeted for prosecution under RICO. Prosecutors favor using RICO because they are able to get convictions with minimal evidence, they are able to combine federal and state offenses, and prison sentences for racketeering are substantially longer than for gambling, drug, and extortion offenses.

According to the RICO statute, racketeering requires a pattern of activity involving two or more "predicates," or distinctly different or isolated offenses that have a common purpose. In other words, the two unrelated, predicate offenses must support the racketeering activity. Examples of predicate offenses are kidnapping and murder in furtherance of a conspiracy to smuggle narcotics.

The state did not have to prove that Dr. Graves criminally prescribed drugs to his patients. They simply paraded about 30 patients who were addicts and were facing prosecution themselves for drug offenses before the jury to testify that they deceived Dr. Graves into illegally prescribing drugs.

The two "predicate" charges against Dr. Graves were drug trafficking (i.e., selling drugs to patients for money) and the manslaughter of patients who died while using the drugs. The interrelated and prejudicial nature of these two charges was acknowledged by the first judge in the Graves' case, Judge Joseph Tarbuck.

Judge Tarbuck said that the charge of drug trafficking had prejudicial "spillover" effect on the charge that Dr. Graves was guilty of manslaughter:

> The jury is very likely to say, if (Dr. Graves) overly prescribed OxyContin to 110 people then he's probably guilty of manslaughter (in the deaths) of patients.[3]

In other words, instead of proving that Dr. Graves was a drug dealer and he was guilty of manslaughter, the racketeering charge implied a connection between the two offenses. Judge Tarbuck later contradicted himself by denying the prejudicial spillover of the two charges after Edgar argued that it would be too costly to Santa Rosa county to hold two trials—one on racketeering and a second on manslaughter. Tarbuck's about-face was fateful and virtually sealed Dr. Graves' fate.

Judge Kenneth Bell replaced Judge Tarbuck just before the trial, for medical reasons. Judge Bell was a politically ambitious judge and was elevated to the Florida Supreme Court following the trial in 2002.

The racketeering charge gave the prosecution a readymade motive. The state did not have to prove beyond a reasonable doubt that Dr. Graves was guilty of selling drugs for money or that his patients died from the drugs he prescribed. It simply presented both predicate offenses as part of a racketeering conspiracy.

Dr. James F. Graves: Indictment and Arrest

On Friday, June 30, 2000, Dr. James F. Graves, a 53-year-old family practitioner for 30 years, was undergoing a heart catherization at Sacred Heart Hospital in Pensacola, Florida, when he learned that a warrant for his arrest had been issued. Alecia Graves, Dr. Graves' wife, phoned her husband's attorney, Dan Stewart, and informed him that several carloads of police from the Santa Rosa Sheriff's office and the Florida Department of Law Enforcement had just arrived at their home to serve an arrest warrant on her husband. *Pensacola News Journal* reporters and a reporter from Channel 3 TV News were also present to cover the arrest of Dr. Graves for broadcast during the normally slow July 4 holiday news weekend.

Assistant State Attorney Russ Edgar, who personally supervised the investigation of Dr. Graves, convened the Santa Rosa County grand jury. Edgar accused Jim Graves of being one of the "biggest drug dealers" in Northeast Florida.[4]

At noon, on Friday, June 30, the grand jury indictment was unsealed. It accused Dr. Graves of four counts of manslaughter, racketeering, drug trafficking, prescribing narcotics to patients without an examination, and exchanging pills for cash. The indictment accused Dr. Graves of distributing thousands of pills to known drug dealers who came to his office as patients or met him in parking lots for cash sales.

When nine police cars arrived at Dr. Graves' home to arrest him, only his 18-year-old daughter Jordan was at home. Frightened, she called her mother, who advised her to go to a friend's house and stay there. Mrs. Graves then contacted Dan Stewart, who proceeded to Sacred Heart Hospital. When Stewart reached the hospital, he learned that Dr. Graves was on a cardiac catherization table with a catheter that entered the femoral artery in the groin leading to his heart. The purpose of catherization is to determine whether a patient has blockage in the coronary arteries and therefore has a risk of heart attack.

Against medical advice, Graves had the catheter removed, applied pressure to his groin to stop the bleeding and got off the table. The standard treatment is for a patient to lie on his back for at least 12 hours before getting up and walking around in order to prevent severe bleeding and potential loss of a limb. He disregarded the danger and went to the Santa Rosa County jail that evening with his attorney where he turned himself into the sheriff. While in his cell, Dr. Graves had bleeding in his groin but was fortunate that he did not suffer more serious medical complications.

James Graves took this unusual risk because he was determined not to be the featured subject of a major media event during the news lull of the Fourth of July weekend. He felt that this would serve only to humiliate him and his family. Graves' bail bond was set at an unprecedented $500,000 at the insistence of the prosecutor, Russ Edgar, on the grounds that "Dr. Graves is one of the biggest drug dealers, and blood money would be used to post bond."[5]

The judge agreed with Edgar's request despite the fact that Dr. Graves was an established member of the community and had lived there with his wife and two children for years. He was unable to raise the bail bond and therefore was forced to stay in jail for three days until the judge lowered the bond to $75,000 on appeal by his attorneys on the grounds that Dr. Graves posed no flight risk and was no danger to himself or the community.

James Graves' Missionary Calling

Dr. Graves was born in Monticello, Kentucky, in 1947. Monticello is a small, poor, rural town of a few thousand in the Appalachia coal mining area of Southeastern Kentucky. His father, Fred Graves, was born in Maine but before settling in Kentucky, he and his brother traveled extensively throughout the South holding Christian revival meetings. His wife Ruth met Fred Graves at a revival meeting and later played the piano at the revivals. Jim Graves grew up in the Immanuel Baptist Church in Monticello. His father was the choir director, and his mother played the organ.

Fred Graves had the first radio and TV business in Monticello. As a boy, Jim Graves helped his father install radio and TV antennas and towers on homes. Later, Fred Graves taught radio and TV repair at the vocational school in nearby Elizabethtown.

Jim Graves was influenced by his maternal grandfather, David Colson Byers, who lived to be 98 years old. David Byers had a mercantile business and bought timber and coal land, which he donated to help establish churches in eastern Kentucky. He served on the town council and was a stalwart of the community.

Jim Graves was also strongly influenced by a local country doctor in Monticello by the name of Mack Roberts. Roberts had a big house on the north end of town. He worked hard in his office all day and then came home and after dinner, saw another 20 or 30 patients who were sitting around on his porch. Roberts delivered many babies for indigent families who lived in the hills around Monticello. He never charged them and often loaded his jeep with groceries and went to their homes to deliver things he knew the families needed. He told them that he was making well baby visits.

This personal, folksy style of medicine appealed to James Graves and became a model for his practice of medicine during and after his service in the Navy. Dr. Graves sought to combine his Christian missionary calling with a career in medicine. He also has always wanted to go on medical missions overseas.

Graves attended the University of Kentucky, where he received a degree in chemistry and then entered the University of Kentucky College of Medicine where he graduated in 1973, with an M.D. Soon after graduating, he went to the Middle East for a three-month surgery preceptorship, working with Drs. Dean Fitzgerald and August Lonegren in Ajiloun, Jordan. He was inspired by their practice of treating ordinary Jordanian citizens in the community.

Upon his return to the States, he went directly to Jackson Memorial Hospital at the University of Miami, where he undertook a one-year surgery internship. He then accepted a demanding three-year surgery residency at Spartanburg General Hospital in South Carolina.

Near the end of his residency, he received a telegram from Dr. George Pael, a Baptist missionary surgeon in Ghana, West Africa. Dr. Peal was the only doctor in the mission hospital that he founded. Pael had a personal medical problem and needed to travel to the United States for treatment. Pael was confronted with a dilemma.

He needed to go to the States for medical treatment, and yet, since he was the only doctor in the clinic, his absence would close down the hospital. He appealed to the International Mission Board (at the time, the Foreign Mission Board) of the Southern Baptist Convention in the United States for a replacement. Graves, who was a member of the Baptist church, agreed to take Dr. Peal's place at the mission hospital while Peal convalesced.

Dr. Graves accepted the missionary assignment. The mission provided little pay but James Graves agreed to put on hold his plans to go into private practice. Within a week's time, Graves and his wife Alecia sold their home, stored their furniture, and went to Ghana to work in the mission hospital.

After Dr. Graves returned to the States in December 1976, he changed his mind about private practice and decided to do public service medicine in the Navy as a flight surgeon. He served for 17 years until he was honorably discharged in 1994. Initially he worked as a *locum tenens* (temporary) doctor under contact with Spectrum, a company that recruited doctors for short-term or replacement positions in hospital emergency rooms in Alabama and Pensacola, Florida.

When Spectrum lost its contracts with the hospitals in the area, Dr. Graves decided to stay in the Pensacola area, which was his duty station during much of his Navy career and where most family friends were. His two teenage children were also enrolled in the local high schools. He worked briefly for the Department of Corrections as a physician and then spent a year and a half working at the Accident and Pain Center, which specialized in treating accident victims. The center was owned by Thomas Hutchins, a chiropractor. Dr. Graves opened his own private practice in September 1998 in Pace, Florida, a small rural country town near Pensacola. The government closed his practice in June 2000.

While in the Navy and in private life, he was inspired by his Christian missionary calling by going on short-term missions in Haiti and Bangalore, India, where he worked with Dr. Rebecca Taylor, a missionary doctor. After Dr. Graves was released on bond in July 2000, and while awaiting his trial in February 2002, he worked at a McDonald's restaurant as a cook and later at Cracker Barrel restaurant as a bus boy and dishwasher to help support his family.[6] In his spare time, he worked without pay as a counselor at the Samaritan's Hands Ministry run by his church, the First Baptist Church of Pensacola. The church provided food, clothing, transportation, medical care, counseling, and paid electric and water bills to prevent the interruption of services for the poor. His job was to interview indigent applicants for assistance and to recommend the amount and form of assistance the church could provide to them.

The first judge assigned to the trial, Judge Joseph Q. Tarbuck, allowed Dr. Graves to leave the state in September 2001, to attend a church seminar in North Carolina despite objections from Russ Edgar that he was a flight risk. Prior to his trial, he planned another foreign medical mission in Kenya, Africa.

A clear indication of Dr. Graves' Christian missionary commitment was that after 30 years of medical practice, he had no income, savings, pensions, or retirement benefits. He was forced to cash in a life insurance policy to post collateral for his bail bond.

In 2001, a court declared Dr. Graves to be indigent and appointed two defense attorneys at the expense of Santa Rosa County. Throughout Dr. Graves' five-week trial, the press kept up a steady drum beat of criticism of the mounting cost of Dr. Graves' defense to Santa Rose County taxpayers. Leading up to and during the trial, the media reported the estimated costs to the public of Dr. Graves' defense. And the prosecutor continued to allege that Graves was bilking the taxpayer because he had money hidden away; illegally obtained from dealing drugs.

For example, the press reported that the public defense of Dr. Graves cost Santa Rosa taxpayers $200,000 before the trial began in January 2002, and $385,000 during the trial.[7] The press reported that this was the most expensive trial in Santa Rosa's history. This angered the public, and the prosecutor used it to inflame public opinion against Dr. Graves and gain national notoriety.

The Criminal Investigation

The criminal investigation of Dr. Graves was set in motion by Dr. Graves' employer, Thomas Hutchins, a chiropractor and owner of the Accident and Pain Clinic where Graves worked from January 1997 until May of 1998. The clinic specialized in postaccident trauma patients, including automobile accident injuries and patients with failed back surgery. The common denominator of these patients was that they were all in some degree of pain.

Hutchins reported Dr. Graves to the Drug Enforcement Agency (DEA) in Pensacola and Tampa in February 1998.[8] Hutchins told the DEA that Dr. Graves was prescribing excessive amounts of narcotic drugs and not recording them in patients' charts, implying nonmedical prescription of drugs. Hutchins also said that Graves met a patient in a parking lot where he took cash in exchange for a prescription of Lortab pills.

Hutchens fired Dr. Graves in May 1998. When he was asked why he discharged Dr. Graves after a year and a half, he said that he discovered that Graves was treating former Accident and Pain Clinic patients at other medical clinics in violation of his "non-compete" contract. Indeed, after Dr. Graves left the clinic, he worked at another clinic in the area owned by Dr. Spain. Hutchins sued both Graves and Spain for violating Graves' noncompete clause in his contract with Hutchins. Hutchins claimed that both doctors were implicated in a conspiracy to harm his business.[9]

According to Graves, the reason Hutchins fired him was that he complained that Hutchins was defrauding the government by up-coding or overbilling the treatment of workers' compensation patients. Shortly after Graves complained,

Hutchins discharged all workers' compensation patients from the clinic and refused to treat them over the objection of Dr. Graves. Indeed, some of these patients followed Dr. Graves when he started his own practice in September 1998. Subsequently, Dr. Graves reported Hutchins for fraudulently billing insurance companies. He even gave depositions to fraud investigators alleging Hutchins' fraudulent billing.[10]

In February 1999, the Tampa diversion unit of the DEA transmitted Tom Hutchins' complaint against Dr. Graves to Special Agent Carl Dennis Norrad of the Florida Department of Law Enforcement (FDLE) in Pensacola. The DEA asked Norrad to take the lead in carrying out a criminal investigation of Dr. Graves.[11] Norrad had a 34-year history of investigating major crimes, including homicides, drug trafficking, and racketeering.

In March 1999, Norrad started gathering evidence against Graves. He talked to a few pharmacists, law enforcement, family members and friends of the overdose victims, and a friend who worked at a funeral home.[12] They said that they were suspicious of Graves' prescriptions and the deaths of his patients.

One pharmacist told Norred that he informed Graves' patients they would die if they continued to take his prescriptions.[13] On March 14, 1999, five months after Dr. Graves opened his practice, one of his patients, Ann Carroll, overdosed and died after being prescribed OxyContin and MS Contin by Dr. Graves two days before her death. Carroll's death rattled some patients and prompted pharmacies to stop filling Dr. Graves' prescriptions.

In August 1999, Norrad officially opened a criminal investigation against Dr. Graves. He said that he had reason to think crimes had occurred and he had a target: Dr. Graves. As the lead investigator or "case agent" representing the DEA's Organized Crime Drug Enforcement Task Force (OCDETF) in North Florida, Norrad represented the DEA's diversion unit, U.S. Defense Criminal Investigative Service, the State Attorney's office, Medicaid Fraud Control Unit of the Agency for Health Care Administration (AHCA), the Santa Rosa and Escambia sheriff's departments, and Florida Department of Insurance.

As the lead investigator, Norrad recruited Sara Lowe, a Pensacola pharmacy oversight fraud inspector for AHCA. AHCA paid for the prescription medications for Medicaid patients. They also kept records of the doctors who prescribed Medicaid patients medications.

Norrad asked Sara Lowe to gather the prescription records of Dr. Graves' patients from October 1998 through March 1999. Norrad also told local police agencies that he wanted to know everything about the drug-overdose deaths of Dr. Graves' patients.

Drug Trafficking

In order to build a criminal case of drug trafficking, Norrad recruited Chris Watson, a detective corporal with the Santa Rosa County Sheriff's Office, narcotics division. Watson's job was to coordinate undercover operations in Dr. Graves' office.

Norrad then enlisted an undercover informant by the name of Paul My-lock. Mylock was a convicted drug felon and addict who was also a patient of Dr. Graves. Mylock made undercover visits to Graves' office on September 20, 1999, October 28, 1999, January 21, 2000, February 10, 2000, and February 24, 2000. These visits constituted the five counts of drug trafficking on which he was tried. Dr. Graves' prescriptions of oxycodone to Mylock, allegedly for no legitimate medical reason, was the state's principal evidence for the racketeering and drug trafficking charges.

Mylock was a 27-year-old pipe wielder and pipefitter by trade with a criminal record of oxycodone addiction. He had three prior felony arrests and convictions for selling cocaine, marijuana, and oxycodone on the street. In May 1999, he was arrested again on drug trafficking charges. At the time of his arrest, Mylock already had federal drug felony conspiracy charges pending against him. If convicted on the prior charges, he could have received up to 25 years in prison. This made Mylock an ideal candidate for an undercover operation against Dr. Graves. Not only was he a patient of Dr. Graves, but Mylock expected to receive credit for his undercover work.

Paul Mylock first went to see Dr. Graves as a patient on June 17, 1999. Even before seeing Dr. Graves, Mylock was addicted to oxycodone, which he bought on the street.[14] He never divulged that fact to Dr. Graves.[15]

Mylock went to see Dr. Graves for back pain and headaches at the suggestion of his stepmother. He saw Dr. Graves on June 17, 1999, soon after he was arrested on drug conspiracy charges in May 26, 1999. Dr. Graves gave Mylock a complete physical exam, including taking his vital signs, monitoring his heart during treadmill exercises, testing leg raises and reflexes.

Mylock told Dr. Graves he had headaches and severe lower back pain due to injury on the job. He also said that he was having trouble sleeping, and reported that his pain level was between 5 and 6 out of a maximum of 10. During the exam, Dr. Graves discovered that Mylock had a markedly irregular pulse and elevated blood pressure. He diagnosed Mylock with high blood pressure, chronic pain, and anxiety.

Dr. Graves prescribed Lopressor to control Mylock's blood pressure, Ambien for sleep, Lortab for short-term (4–6 hours) pain relief, and Xanax to relieve tension. Graves refused to give Mylock anything for his long-term chronic back pain until he checked it out. Dr. Graves told Mylock that he wanted him to first see Dr. Cherian, a local cardiologist in Milton, to have a Holter monitor test, which records heart rhythm over a 24-hour period. He also told Mylock to have an X-ray of his back. Mylock ignored Graves' instructions and told him that he was trying to schedule the tests.

On July 2, and July 20, 1999, Mylock made his scheduled follow-up visits, and each time, his vital signs were taken. On July 20, Mylock was first prescribed OxyContin in the relatively low 20 mg. strength. This was in response to his continued complaint of back pain and headaches.[16] Mylock never told Dr. Graves that he had used OxyContin before.

The only drug prescribed by Dr. Graves that Mylock actually took was Lortab (hydrocodone) and OxyContin. Furthermore, he did not take them as

Graves directed but rather chewed the tablets and added to the dosage by illegally buying OxyContin pills off the street and eating them.

The Undercover Operation

On September 14, 1999, Mylock accepted Russ Edgar's offer to become an undercover agent, and on September 20th, Mylock visited Dr. Graves for the first time wearing a recording device. He was under the supervision of Dennis Norrad and Detective Chris Watson. Mylock was sent into Graves' office a total of five times from September 20, 1999 till February 24, 2000. The last three times were at the request of the prosecutor, Russ Edgar. Mylock visited Dr. Graves on his own without a wire and without informing law enforcement in November 1999, in order to get a prescription for OxyContin, which he took.

On the September 20, 1999 visit, Mylock again complained about his back pain and headaches. He said that he took a couple of his stepmother's Soma (muscle relaxer) tablets and this gave him some relief. Dr. Graves told him he had scheduled an appointment for him with a cardiologist. Dr. Graves prescribed Lopressor, Lortabs, Vioxx, Soma, and OxyContin 40 mg. twice a day for his chronic back pain. Mylock missed his next scheduled appointment on October 18, 1999, but returned on October 28, 1999, wearing his recording device.

During that visit, Mylock apologized because he had not taken the Holter monitor test. Dr. Graves said that he was concerned about Mylock's elevated heart rate. He warned him not to miss appointments and not to run out of his medication. Graves stressed that Mylock should continue to take Lopressor and treat his pain in order to keep his heart rate down.[17]

Mylock missed his December appointment with Graves and went to his office on January 21, 2000. He explained that he missed the last appointment because he was working out of town. Mylock asked for steroids, but Dr. Graves refused telling him to buy over-the-counter vitamins instead. Graves also told Mylock he wanted him to take an EKG for his heart as soon as his new machine arrived. Graves prescribed Lortab for short-term "breakthrough pain," Soma, Vioxx, Norvasc, Xanax, Lopressor, and one OxyContin 80 mg tablet at night for chronic pain relief.

Mylock returned to Dr. Graves' office on February 10, 2000, four days before his regularly scheduled appointment. He said that he had taken more OxyContin than Graves had prescribed because of the pain. Mylock said that he ran out of the 40 mg tablets and took three 80 mg tablets a day. Graves warned Mylock against taking such a high dosage. Dr. Graves told him to take two 40 mg tablets at intervals during the day and only one 80 mg table at night for pain relief.

Mylock complained to Dr. Graves about the difficulty he was having with his construction job in Mississippi and asked about a new career as an Excel telephone representative. Graves had a banner in the office advertising that he was an Excel representative. Mylock asked Dr. Graves for help in becoming a phone representative.

Mylock's next visit to Dr. Graves' office was on February 24, 1999. It was also unscheduled. Russ Edgar highlighted to the jury Mylock's recording of this visit. At Edgar's direction, Mylock went to Dr. Graves' office for the purpose of signing up as an Excel telephone representative. Edgar gave him $250 dollars for the start-up costs of the Excel program and the training kit. Graves took the money and mailed his personal check to Excel for that amount. Graves told Mylock to make an appointment with him for training after the Excel kit arrived in the mail.

Near the end of the meeting, Mylock told Dr. Graves that he would be out of town for the next three weeks in Mississippi and therefore would be unable to make his regularly scheduled visit on March 9. He said that his daughter was having oral surgery the next day and he wanted to spend time with his family instead of returning from Mississippi to pick up another prescription. Mylock asked if Dr. Graves would give him his prescriptions early; he was willing to pay Dr. Graves $60 for the prescription appointment plus $25 for the early prescriptions, the normal office charge.

Dr. Graves checked Mylock's chart before writing the prescriptions. He told Mylock that he wanted to ensure that he had enough blood pressure medications. He gave him OcyContin, Lortab, Soma, and Vioxx early and said that it was just a matter of managing his pain medication so that he did not run out. Dr. Graves told him which pills to take and how often to take them. He also discussed the least expensive dosage of OxyContin tablets to take pointing out that it was less expensive to take two 20 mg tablets than one 40 mg. Graves said the price discrepancy was ridiculous.

The Prosecutor Goes Undercover

By January 2000, Dennis Norrad persuaded the State Attorney's Office to prosecute Dr. Graves. Norrad claimed that Graves was "hooking" patients on deadly narcotic prescriptions. He argued that if Graves were allowed to continue prescribing narcotics, it would lead to additional overdose deaths.

The deaths of Gwen Carpenter on December 21, 1999, and Howard Rice on April 12, 2000, accelerated the investigation. Edgar described the case as a race for time with two goals. The first was to stop James Graves' "criminal activity" and the resulting overdose deaths. The second was to ensure that Edgar had a prosecutable criminal case.

To that end, Edgar instructed Norrad to order Mylock to make three more undercover visits to Graves' office. Edgar also carried out his own undercover operation on February 4, 2000. He and Special Agent Haley interviewed Dr. Graves in his office. They secretly wired themselves for the interview for later use in Graves' trial

The events leading to the interview were that Dr. Graves wrote a letter to the State Attorney's Office on January 31, 2000, asking to meet with a representative. He did this after a pharmacist contacted him to report that Sara Lowe, the Medicaid pharmacy fraud investigator, faxed a request for Dr. Graves' prescription records.

The meeting in Dr. Graves' office lasted about one hour. During the interview, Dr. Graves expressed concern that some patients were diverting his prescription drugs and gave Edgar a list of patients he suspected. Edgar and Haley asked Dr. Graves if he could detect addicts who were doctor-shopping for narcotics.[18]

Graves said that sometimes he could. When asked how he could, Dr. Graves said that he looked for needle tracks or marks on their bodies. Graves said that if he saw evidence of needle marks, he "launch(ed) them right out the door."[19]

After the meeting, Edgar and Haley set about refuting Dr. Graves' claim by using drug felons among his patients in undercover operations. They recruited Martha Blackmon, who had needle marks from injecting drugs and who also had received narcotics prescriptions from Dr. Graves.[20]

Martha Blackmon and her husband, Danny Blackmon, were a young couple with three small children. They had an electrical business, and Danny was the electrician. They were injured in a car crash, and Danny Blackmon had work-related injuries. They both had drug dependency problems but worked and cared for their children. Dr. Graves noticed that they had needle marks on their arms. He confronted them separately about misusing the drugs after meeting them a couple of times. They acknowledged that they had a dependency problem, and he scheduled them for evaluation and possible admission to a drug rehabilitation facility at West Florida Hospital. Graves wanted them to go through the treatment one at a time, for 28 days each, with the other remaining home to take care of the children. Martha Blackmon went to register for the program, but Danny did not go because he was arrested on DUI charges after a car crash.

Martha was desperate to get her husband out of jail, so she agreed to wear a wire into Graves' office after Edgar promised her husband leniency by letting Danny off with little or no jail time. During the undercover office visit, Dr. Graves warned Martha not to inject the drugs he had prescribed for her chronic pain. He reluctantly agreed to write her prescriptions to treat the pain until she entered a drug rehabilitation program. Graves did this because she had young children and her husband was in jail, so there was no one to look after them.[21] At the trial, the prosecution sought to impeach Dr. Graves' recorded statement to Edgar and Haley that if he saw needle marks on patients' arms, he "launched them out the door." They did this by playing Martha Blackmon's recording of her office visit in which Dr. Graves warned her not to inject the drugs but gave her a prescription until she entered drug rehabilitation.

Dr. Graves subsequently terminated Martha and Danny when they failed to follow through with the rehabilitation plan.[22] The tragedy was that neither Martha nor Danny received the drug rehabilitation they needed, and two and a half years after Dr. Graves was sent to jail, both of them died of drug overdoses.

Medical Manslaughter: Criminalizing Malpractice

Dr. Graves was charged with manslaughter by "culpable negligence" in the deaths of four patients: Jeffrey Daniels, Gwen Carpenter, Howard Rice, and William Morris. He was accused of illegally prescribing drugs "not in good faith or in the course of his professional practice as a physician," which caused the death of the patients.

In order to support the charge of manslaughter, the prosecution substituted the legal standards for malpractice, which is a civil offense, for the criminal offense of manslaughter. In other words, the prosecution criminalized malpractice in the Graves case.

Medical malpractice is carelessness by a physician that results in injures or death of a patient. It is no different in theory from carelessness by a motorist who does not pay attention to his driving, runs a red light, and causes an injury. Examples of malpractice resulting in death include a physician's failing to control a patient's diabetes who subsequently dies from a diabetic coma.

The most common legal basis for malpractice suits are doctors who do not follow the so-called "standard of care" or conventional treatment therapy that physicians would have followed in a similar situation. If a physician does not follow treatment protocols that at least a "respectable minority" of doctors would have followed, and the patient is injured or dies as a result, it is malpractice. In other words, standard of care is a treatment practiced by some doctors even if it is not the most popular one. In most medical malpractice cases, the testimony of physicians is required to determine whether a breach in the standard of care occurred. In other words, expert medical testimony, not the opinion of a lay jury, is necessary to judge whether malpractice has occurred.

Manslaughter, on the other hand, is accidentally causing unlawful death. It can occur in the heat of passion as when a battered wife kills her violent husband trying to defend herself, or it can occur as a result of "culpable negligence." Death by culpable negligence occurs when an action that a *reasonable person* would not have taken results in death. An example of this is fans at a football game setting off a flare that does not rise in the air as expected, but strikes and kills a person in the stands. This is an accidental death resulting from reckless behavior that a reasonable person would not have taken. In Dr. Graves' case, in order to be found guilty of manslaughter by culpable negligence, the state would have to prove that he was guilty of reckless acts and that his action was the cause of his patients' deaths.

The State's Failure to Prove Manslaughter

The prosecution relied upon the testimony of two expert witnesses, Dr. David Brown and Dr. Theodore V. Parran, to prove that Dr. Graves was guilty of manslaughter. For example, after Dr. Brown reviewed James Graves' patient and pharmacy records and statements of family and friends, he used malpractice standards in concluding that Graves' treatment of his deceased patients "seemed to be outside the bounds of standard medical care."[23] Dr. Parran also testified that Dr. Graves prescribed narcotic pain medication "outside the accepted medical care."[24]

Neither prosecution witness testified that Dr. Graves' acts were wanton, reckless, totally inappropriate, grievously unreasonable, grossly incompetent or purposely homicidal. They also did not testify that Dr. Graves acted as a drug dealer for profit or that the drugs he prescribed were the cause of patients' deaths. Furthermore, their opinion that James Graves prescribed drugs outside the bounds of standard medical care was challenged by two equally qualified physicians.

Dr. Daniel Handel and Dr. Ethan Loucks testified for the defense that Dr. Graves' treatment of the deceased patients was within the standard of care in the United States and was for a legitimate medical purpose.[25] Malpractice lawsuits with clashing expert opinions about standard of care usually fail. However, in a criminal case, evidence must be proven by a higher standard of reasonable doubt. Contradictory opinions expressed by equally qualified expert witnesses clearly do not meet that standard.

Manslaughter by culpable negligence in Section 782.07 Florida statutes requires proof that a defendant's actions are both culpably negligent and the cause of the alleged victims' death. The prosecution failed to prove that Dr. Graves was culpably negligent, but it also failed to prove that he was the cause of his patients' deaths.

For example, in the case of patient Jeffrey Daniels, who died November 10, 1999, the testimony of Dr. Gary Cumberland, M.D., the physician who did the autopsy of Daniels, concluded that he died from an accidental drug overdose.[26] Against Dr. Graves' advice and knowledge, Daniels took alcohol as well as Xanax, some of which he got from his roommate.

In the case of Gwen Carpenter who died on December 21, 1999 of an accidental overdose of drugs, Dr. Cumberland's autopsy found her death was due to a lethal combination of drugs she took.[27] Carpenter took narcotics from her sister and aunt that they had obtained from Dr. Graves by lying about their medical condition. Dr. Graves had no knowledge that Carpenter was getting narcotics from others. He also carefully monitored and limited the narcotics prescriptions. For example, shortly before her death, she went to Dr. Graves' office to get pain medication before her scheduled visit and was refused. Graves injected her with a nonnarcotic pain medication and told her to go to the emergency room of the hospital for evaluation.

Howard Rice died on April 12, 2000 due to an accidental overdose of drugs. He had HIV, depression, and a history of suicide attempts. Rice had one leg shorter than the other and suffered from hip and lower back pain. Dr. Graves ordered an MRI test that revealed a slippage of one vertebra forward on another, which caused chronic pain. Another doctor treated Rice for his HIV but refused to treat his pain on the grounds that Rice had twice attempted suicide. The doctor did not inform Dr. Graves that Howard Rice was a suicide risk. In the end, Rice injected the pain medication Dr. Graves had prescribed instead of taking it as instructed, overdosed, and died.

William Morris also caused his own death on June 28, 2000. Against Dr. Graves' instructions, Morris crushed an OxyContin prescription, mixed it with water, and injected a large quantity into his body, resulting in death.

Spurious Evidence for Manslaughter

The prosecution's evidence against Dr. Graves for manslaughter was based largely upon nonmedical testimony gathered from pharmacists and the families and friends of the deceased patients. Dennis Norrad, Corporal Watson, and another special agent with the Florida Department of Law Enforcement, Dennis Haley, interviewed the pharmacists who filled Dr. Graves' prescriptions for the deceased, family members and friends. The detectives asked for their opinions about the consequences of taking Dr. Graves' prescription drugs.

For example, Thomas Weekly, the owner of Weekly's Pharmacy, told Agent Haley that the OxyContin Dr. Graves prescribed for patients with "back pain" was inappropriate because OxyContin was only designed for "terminally ill" cancer patients.[28] Lawrence Chastain, another pharmacist at K-Mart, said that Dr. Graves "prescribes too many and too much drugs to his patients" and prescribes "the same heavy narcotics." He referred to his prescriptions as "Graves' Cocktail."

Marilyn Earnhardt, a pharmacist at Wal-Mart Pharmacy in Milton, Florida, told Detective Haley and Corporal Watson that patients who had prescriptions from Dr. Graves did not appear to be the usual recipients of powerful narcotics—"terminally ill cancer patients"—instead they appeared to be "street users."[29] Pharmacists also reported that Graves' Cocktails had a lethal effect on patients and were given to drug addicts.

Interviews with the relatives and friends of patients who died reinforced the opinions of the pharmacists. For example, Shane Carroll, the son of Anne Carroll, said that when his mother went to visit Dr. Graves, she was "staggering, obviously intoxicated."[30] Jane Daniels, the mother of Jeffrey Daniels who was a patient of Dr. Graves and fatally overdosed in November 1999, accused Graves of killing her son.[31]

This made it relatively easy for the prosecution to infer a connection between Graves' prescriptions and homicide. To support his theory of homicide, Edgar created a timeline for the overdose deaths of Graves' patients. He listed seven patients who died in 1999, six in 2000, and three in 2001. Examination of the list of overdose deaths, however, does not support the prosecution's claim that they received narcotic prescriptions from Dr. Graves or, indeed, that they were even his patients.[32]

Investigators also interviewed convicted felons who were in the Santa Rosa and Escambia county jails. They were addicts, and some were both pain patients and drug dealers who scammed Dr. Graves into writing prescription narcotics for them. Indeed, at Graves' trial, dozens of addicts who tricked

Dr. Graves into giving them narcotic prescriptions testified against him in court in return for lighter sentences.

Devastation to the Graves Family

After the jury convicted Dr. Graves on February 19, 2002, Judge Kenneth B. Bell imposed an unprecedented life sentence on Dr. Graves. He was given more than 62 years in prison. After Dr. Graves was tried and sent to jail, his wife, Alecia, and their teenage daughter, Jordan, were forced to move from a home they were renting for about $1,000 per month. Alecia Graves found employment at Hallmark Elementary School in Escambia County, teaching first grade. She also took a second job as a sales clerk at Victoria Secrets on weekends and holidays.

At the time of Dr. Graves' trial, his 22-year-old son, Jimmy, was majoring in chemical engineering at the University of Alabama. After Dr. Graves' practice was shut down in April 2000, Jimmy's support ended, and he got a job working 35 hours a week, delivering food from restaurants during the lunch and evening shifts as a driver while completing his education. After college, he obtained a job with Eastman Chemical Company in Texas. While in college and since, Jimmy Graves has supported himself and helped support his mother. For example, he signed a lease for his mother to rent a condo in Pensacola at $670 per month so that she could be near her work.

In the summer of 2002, Jimmy's sister, Jordan, left Milton, Florida, to attend the University of Florida in Gainsville. She was a straight "A" student and received a state scholarship, plus the cost of books. She also has a job to support herself while completing a course of study in the school of nursing. The trauma of the ordeal was such that, to this day, she refuses to discuss it.

DR. FRANK B. FISHER: SOCIAL JUSTICE FOR THE POOR

On the morning of February 18, 1999, more than 20 heavily armed officers from several law enforcement agencies swarmed into the clinic of Dr. Frank Bensell Fisher, M.D., in Anderson, California, just south of Redding. A simultaneous raid was carried out seven miles away at the Shasta Pharmacy in Redding, which was owned and operated by Stephen Miller, the pharmacist, and Madeline Miller, his wife and pharmacy manager.

Dr. Fisher and the Millers were handcuffed and taken to jail. Fisher's bank account was seized, and his bail was set at $15 million. This is greater than the bail set for Colombian drug lords. He could not make bail and was forced to spend five months in the Shasta County Jail during the preliminary hearings of his trial. The Millers' bank accounts were also seized, and their bail was set at $3 million each. They were also unable to make bail and were jailed for five months. Employees of the clinic and pharmacy were detained, the buildings were searched, their computers were seized, and office records were boxed and taken away by the police.

Dr. Fisher and the Millers were charged with murder, distributing narcotics illegally, and defrauding the state of California. Bill Lockyer, the California Attorney General, had been in office for about one month before he held a press conference in Redding to announce the arrest. He declared that Dr. Fisher and the Millers were part of a "highly sophisticated drug-dealing operation" that caused the overdose deaths of at least three people, addicted hundreds of others who became "hooked on narcotics," and bilked Medi-Cal out of $2 million.[33] Lockyer said that this was the biggest drug ring in the history of Northern California. The Attorney General elaborated,

We are shutting down suppliers of a highly addictive drug (*Oxycontin*) that has been improperly allowed to saturate the community. Dr. Fisher was operating a patient mill, prescribing controlled drugs after superficial examinations and then submitting billings to Medi-Cal.[34]

Gary A. Binkard, The deputy Attorney General, who was in office before Lockyear was elected, was the chief prosecutor in the case. He declared:

The facts in this case suggest that this trio of individuals are more akin to a person who poisoned a county well and caused the deaths of the people who were unfortunate enough to drink from it.[35]

Binkerd compared Dr. Fisher and the Millers to common "street pushers" whose sole interest was to pump out "staggering quantities of pain medicine."[36] Prosecutors claimed that Dr. Fisher prescribed massive amounts of narcotics to patients and then sent them to the Shasta Pharmacy where the owners, Stephen and Madeline Miller, filled the prescriptions.

According to the government, Frank Fisher and the Millers created a "public health epidemic with attendant abuse, addiction, overdose and death."[37] Anthony Lewis, a prosecutor in the Attorney General's Office, said that Fisher's clinic was a "nefarious and dangerous pill mill" and the Millers distributed drugs in a "candy store" fashion.

Frank Fisher's Indian Heritage

In order to understand why the government targeted Dr. Fisher for prosecution, it is necessary to understand his family background and upbringing. Frank Fisher grew up in the 1950s with his mother and father and one brother in Berkeley, California. His father, Frank Fisher, Sr., was a medical corpsman in the Navy during WW II. After the war, he attended Lewis and Clark College in Oregon to become a teacher. He was the first generation in his family to go to college. After graduation, he got a job teaching high school in Oakland, California. Frank Fisher, Sr., met his wife, Joan, in college where she was also training to be a teacher. She graduated and was credentialed to teach but decided instead to work as a housewife and raise her two sons.

Joan Fisher was a member of the Confederation Tribes of Siletz Indians in Oregon. This is a confederation of 27 tribal bands that once inhabited a range from northern California to southwest Washington. The Confederation took its name from the Siletz river in Oregon where the U.S. Army relocated them on a reservation during the 1850s. The Siletz Reservation now contains 3,838 acres of Oregon Coast Range timberland. It has a tribal population of about 4,000 scattered throughout an 11-county area of western Oregon.

In 1851, the federal government forced 2,025 Indians of various tribes onto the reservation at Siletz. Only 259 of the Indians had treaties with the U.S. Congress. About 760 Indians did not qualify for assistance from the government. This resulted in a dramatic decline in their health and welfare. The Siletz Indians were forced to adopt "white ways" on the reservations.[38] This resulted in a complete breakdown of the indigenous social and economic structures and led to a miserable and impoverished life on the Siletz reservation.

In 1989, a family of three with a cash income below $9,885 was defined as living in poverty, and 27 percent of all American Indian families lived below this poverty level.[39] American Indians have the poorest health in the country. American Indians and Alaska Natives born in 2002 have a life expectancy of almost six years less than the U.S. average. Death rates due to alcoholism are 7.7 times greater, tuberculosis is 7.5 times higher, diabetes 4.2 times greater, accidents 2.8 times greater, homicide 2.1 times higher, and unsanitary water and waste disposal facilities are 7.5 higher for American Indian homes. The 2003 U.S. Commission on Civil Rights reported that American Indians suffer from a "quiet crisis" of poverty, unemployment, substance abuse, school dropout, and epidemic levels of diabetes, cancer, and heart disease.[40]

As a boy, Frank Fisher spent his summers at the Siletz Reservation with his maternal grandfather, Art Bensell and grandmother, Margaret Bensell. They owned the general store, and Art Bensell was the mayor of the town of about 500 residents. He was the town butcher and worked 14-hour days. Unlike other Siletz Indians who were forced to sell their land to survive, Art Bensell retained ownership of his land. He later became the Siletz tribal chairman, knew everyone on the reservation and had personal ties with political leaders in Oregon, including U.S. Senator Mark Hatfield. Art Bensell's concern for his people was evident during the 1980s, when he established a substance abuse program for tribal members and managed it.

During Frank Fisher's visits to Siletz, he got to know fellow tribal members and became familiar with their culture of poverty and the health crisis confronting them. This experience left a lasting impression on him. He and his brother continued their membership in the Siletz Confederation of Tribes. His brother became an attorney and assumed the position of tribal judge with the Confederated Tribes of Siletz.

Harvard Medical School and the Indian Health Service

During the mid-1970s, Harvard Medical School adopted a policy of diversifying its student body by enrolling students from underprivileged backgrounds.

Harvard's expectation was that these students would return to serve their destitute communities after graduation.

Frank Fisher was recruited because of his Indian background. In his case, the plan worked because after graduating from medical school and completing an internship at Saint Mary's Hospital in San Francisco in 1982, he went to work for the Indian Health Service. This is the only government health service that is rated below the Bureau of Indian Affairs.

For the next 10 years, he worked at over 20 Indian reservations throughout the Midwest and Western United States. He moved from one Indian clinic or hospital after another as needed, providing desperately needed health care spending a few months at each reservation. There was always a dire shortage of doctors on Indian reservations because they are remote, poverty is extreme, and the pay is the lowest that a physician can make.

Frank Fisher began working at the Yankton Sioux tribe reservation in Wagner, South Dakota. He was paid just over $7 dollars an hour. During the next 10 years working on reservations, he averaged between $100 and $150 per day plus housing and hospital or clinic food. His work was rewarded in other ways, however. Foremost among them, he knew his services were needed and appreciated. Despite that, Dr. Fisher was never able to save for his future retirement. He had been working in Indian clinics and emergency hospital rooms and was never motivated to make much money.

In 1990, he decided to move back to the San Francisco area to be closer to his aging parents, settle down, and build economic security for retirement. Initially, he worked at Indian reservations in California, and then in inner city clinics as a *locum tenens* in San Francisco, Oakland, and San Jose that mostly served Indians and the impoverished who were on federal Medicaid, called Medi-Cal in California. He felt comfortable in this culture.

With his Indian background, he was uniquely able to understand and treat their medical problems. He understood, for example, that poor people seek medical treatment for survival issues, not for prevention or "life style" concerns. For example, they want antibiotics to treat infections, not cholesterol-lowering drugs. Being overweight was not their worry. Frank Fisher related one experience in which white doctors working at a reservation clinic prescribed cholesterol drugs to Indians. When Dr. Fisher left the clinic at the end of the day, he found pill bottles containing the drugs scattered all over the grounds of the clinic.

During the 1990s, Dr. Fisher set up his own community clinic called the Westwood Walk-in Clinic in Anderson, California. Between 80 and 90 percent of his patients were Indian and poor. About 80 percent of his patients were on Medi-Cal, 10 percent were on Medicare, 5 percent were on private insurance, and 5 percent were poor, cash-paying patients.

Compassionate Medicine

Dr. Fisher was placed in a risky situation that all physicians fear when treating patients with chronic pain. It is a dilemma between a desire to practice compassionate medicine and the awareness that to do so may not be tolerated by law enforcement authorities. Despite the danger, experiences in his personal and professional life led him to choose compassionate medicine. Dr. Fisher's father, Frank Fisher, Sr., was a medical corpsman in the Navy during WW II. He told Frank, Jr., about an experience in which he accidentally administered 10 times as much morphine to a wounded sailor as the doctor had prescribed. Concerned about the dosage, Frank, Sr., observed the patient carefully for the next few hours. He was surprised to discover that the patient's behavior changed dramatically for the better. He was able to get out of bed and go to the bathroom by himself, something that he previously needed assistance to do. When the dose wore off, however, the sailor was once again in great pain and was unable to get out of bed.

Frank Fisher, Jr., also had a personal experience using narcotics to relieve pain. On the day that he was scheduled to be interviewed for admission to Harvard Medical School, the muscles in his back went into painful spasm. He went to the University of California Health Services center where a doctor prescribed Tylenol #3, which contains codeine (opium) and Valium.

The doctor told Frank, Jr., that it was necessary to take Tylenol and Valium in combination to break the pain cycle. Valium was needed to relieve the muscle spasms by relaxing the muscles, and codeine was necessary to treat the pain directly. The doctor gave Fisher between 20 and 30 pills of Valium and Tylenol #3, which he used over the next few years during medical school to relieve his back pain. This experience made him understand the reinforcing nature of pain and instilled the belief that the combination of opioids and muscle relaxers was a safe and effective treatment for relief. The question of addiction never arose.

Dr. Fisher's training at Harvard also encouraged him to practice compassionate medicine. For example, during his rotation through orthopedic surgery at Massachusetts General Hospital (MGH), he received instruction from Dr. Hugh Chandler who performed the first hip replacement in the United States. All of Chandler's patients were pain sufferers whom he treated with opioids to relieve their pain. This reinforced the idea in Fisher's mind that opioids were an appropriate, safe, and effective way to manage pain. He learned from Chandler the importance of increasing the dosages of opioids (called titration) until a patient receives relief from his pain.

Dr. Fisher also learned the "customer approach to patienthood" taught at Harvard. Dr. John Stoeckle, the director of the primary care unit at MGH, taught him that in order to treat a patient, it is necessary to find out what his agenda or goals are for treatment. Dr. Leston Havens, his teacher of psychiatry at Harvard, also taught him the empathic interview method of treatment that requires a doctor to listen to his own feelings in order to tune into what a patient is experiencing.

The effect of his personal experience with narcotics and his training at Harvard left a lasting impression upon him. For the next 20 years of practice, he felt like an imposter practicing medicine whenever he told a patient who was experiencing severe chronic pain that he would have to "learn to live with it" because there was nothing he could do for him.

The California Pain Patient's Bill of Rights

The passage of the California Pain Patient's Bill of Rights in 1997 changed all that. For the first time, Dr. Fisher felt that he could practice compassionate medicine. The bill authorized doctors to treat patients suffering from Chronic Intractable Pain (CIP) with the necessary narcotics to relieve their pain. The Act removed Dr. Fisher's fear of prescribing narcotics to pain patients.

Furthermore, since Fisher had been under fraud investigation for prescribing the opiate, Vicodin, and the muscle-relaxer, Soma (similar to the codine/Valium combination Fisher had earlier used with success on himself), he decided to follow the guidelines of the Chronic Pain Bill and increase rather than decrease the dosage of pain medication to relieve patients' suffering. Instead of making it more secure for Dr. Fisher to prescribe narcotics, it virtually guaranteed his prosecution. The reason was that law enforcement agents interpreted Dr. Fisher's actions as deliberately provocative and a challenge to their authority.

Soon after the bill was passed, a representative of Purdue Pharma, the manufacturer of OxyContin, contacted Dr. Fisher and told him about their new "miracle" pain relief medication. Frank Fisher was keenly interested in the drug and sought to acquire more knowledge about its use and the use of opioids in general, to relieve pain suffers. He attended a conference on chronic pain control in Concord, California, in the Fall of 1998, and joined the American Pain Society, the oldest pain association in the country.

Armed with the illusion of legal protection and powerful new pain relief drugs, Dr. Fisher started prescribing sizeable doses of narcotics to his chronic pain patients. Consequently, there was a large jump in Fisher's prescriptions of narcotics in 1998. At the time of his arrest in February 1999, Dr. Fisher had about 3,000 patients. Between 5 and 10 percent of them (i.e., 150 and 300) were chronic pain sufferers. Between 10 and 15 of his patients were on high doses of OxyContin, with another 30 patients on lower doses of the drug.

The government used the growth in the volume of narcotics prescribed by Dr. Fisher and dispensed by the Shasta Pharmacy as evidence of a conspiracy. Joyce Rutan, the pharmacy chief of Medi-Cal for Northern California, testified that Dr. Fisher prescribed over $1,000,000 worth of OxyContin in 1998. This was an expensive pain medication that cost the state as much as $8.00 a pill. She said that according to the DEA, Shasta Pharmacy was the top purchaser of OxyContin in California. For example during 1998, Shasta purchased 14,336 grams of OxyContin. She also said that Dr. Fisher was the top prescriber of OxyContin out of 50,000 doctors in the state of California and proclaimed that Dr. Fisher and the Millers thus constituted a public health hazard that constituted an epidemic.

The problem with Rutan's claim is that the government's own expert witness, Dr. John Eisele, testified that Frank Fisher's narcotics prescriptions to CIP patients was perfectly normal and Eisele had himself prescribed much higher doses of opioids to pain patients. For example, a difficult pain patient might require between three or four grams of OxyContin per day times 365 days, which would be between 1,950 and 1,460 grams per year. Dr. Fisher reported that he had about 10 CIP patients requiring high doses of OxyContin. That would be close to the 14,336 grams that Dr. Fisher prescribed and Shasta dispensed in 1998.[41]

Madeline Miller: A Pain Patient Advocate

Frank Fisher and the Millers were arrested on February 18, 1999, less than three months after Madeline Miller successfully challenged Medi-Cal's refusal to pay for the medications of one of Dr. Fisher's indigent pain patients on February 3. That was the date that a state administrative law judge ordered Medi-Cal to pay Shasta Pharmacy for the pain prescriptions for one of Dr. Fisher's patients. In issuing the ruling, the administrative law judge commended Dr. Fisher and the Millers for keeping accurate records and ordered Medi-Cal to pay for the patient's medication. This set a legal precedent for about 100 additional cases involving Dr. Fisher that Medi-Cal had also refused to pay.[42] Indeed, mass hearings for about 80 additional cases were scheduled for April 7–9, 1999.

Magdeline Miller's activist role on behalf of indigent pain patients undoubtedly played a part in the government's decision to prosecute the Millers and Dr. Fisher. Mrs. Miller decided to challenge Medi-Cal for two reasons. The first was that she was one of Frank Fisher's pain patients. She suffered from a crippling back injury and Attention Deficit Disorder and, therefore, understood the plight of chronic pain sufferers. Miller believed in the American principle of guaranteeing social justice to poor people by legally empowering them to enforce their rights to public housing, food stamps, welfare benefits, and health care through the courts. According to the federal Medicaid Act, an individual is entitled to Medicaid benefits if he meets the criteria established by the state in which he lives.[43] For example, in *Frank v. Kizer 1990*, the state supreme court ruled that Medi-Cal must provide "Aid Paid Pending" and not cut off any Medi-Cal recipient from his medicine until he was given a fair hearing.[44] This ruling, along with the pain Act, gave Miller the legal ammunition to force Medi-Cal to approve medication claims on behalf of pain patients.

Madeline Miller and her husband, the pharmacist and owner of Shasta Pharmacy, refused to turn Dr. Fisher's pain patients away without dispensing their medications, whether Medi-Cal authorized payment or not. In fact, the Millers continued to dispense pain medication to indigent Medi-Cal patients at their own expense until they could resolve the payment issue with Medi-Cal.

Just before their arrest on February 18, they had spent about $40,000 of their own money to pay for indigents' prescriptions until they could be reimbursed by Medi-Cal. They kept a log book of out-of-pocket expenses to pay for the medications. The Millers felt they had a moral responsibility to ensure that chronic pain patients received their medications. In late 1998, Dr. Fisher learned that the Millers were covering the cost of his indigent patients' medications and offered to share the burden if it became too onerous for them to bear. This put a lie to the government's claim that Dr. Fisher and the Miller's were in a conspiracy to defraud the Medi-Cal program.

Madeline Miller was outraged that Joyce Rutan, the head of the Northern Pharmacy Section, or sometimes referred to as the Stockton Medical drug unit, that approved Medi-Cal payments for drug prescriptions in Northern California, was breaking the law by not approving payments for pain medication for Dr. Fisher's patients.

Miller's attorney filed a complaint on behalf of one of Dr. Fisher's pain patients, which was heard on January 20, 1999. The judge who heard the case ruled on February 3, 1999 that Medi-Cal had violated the Chronic Intractable Pain Act and ignored the 1990 state supreme court ruling in *Frank v. Kizer* that ordered Medi-Cal to give patients "Aid Paid Pending" and not cut off any Medi-Cal recipient from his medicine until he was given a fair hearing.[45]

Patient Advocacy Becomes Criminal Conspiracy

The event that triggered the arrest of Frank Fisher and the Millers was a two-hour meeting on October 20, 1998 at the office of Senator Leroy Greene, the author of the Chronic Pain Act. It included Dr. Fisher, Madeline Miller and their attorney, Mark Merin, and Joyce Rutan, the chief of the Stockton Medical drug unit and Rutan's supervisor. Magdeline Miller had asked Senator Greene to call the meeting in order to protest Medi-Cal's denial of payments to Shasta Pharmacy for Dr. Fisher's pain patients. Greene was angered to learn of the government's denial of payment for pain medication because of his personal experience. During the 1980s, Senator Greene's wife became terminally ill with cancer and suffered unnecessarily because she was not given sufficient pain medication to ease her suffering. Indeed, this was the driving force behind Greene's sponsorship of the Chronic Pain Bill in 1997.

Joyce Rutan said she was shocked by the presence of Dr. Fisher and an attorney at the meeting. She was also highly offended by comments made to her at the meeting by Senator Greene and Madeline Miller. For example, Senator Greene demanded to know why Rutan's department was refusing to pay for the pain medications of Medi-Cal patients and said, "Are you aware that you are breaking the law, girlie?"[46] Rutan described Madeline Miller's behavior at the meeting as "very aggressive, very upsett(ing) and very excitable."[47] She said that Miller used abusive language similar to previous remarks she had made to Rutan in "harassing phone calls to her office."[48]

At the meeting, Miller had a "big tub" of Treatment Authorization Requests (TARs) to pay for patient medications that Rutan's department had denied or deferred. The significance of the TARs is that in California, doctors can only prescribe narcotic medications to Medi-Cal patients on special prescription pads that are issued by the state; they are called "triplicates." Doctors are entitled to only 100 triplicates a month. If they need more, they must apply for additional monthly triplicates.

In Dr. Fisher's case, after months of arguing with the State, he was able to obtain only 200 triplicates per month. That was not enough to treat all of his chronic pain patients, which were as many as 400 or about 10 percent of this entire patient population. His only solution short of refusing medication for pain patients was for him to increase the prescription pill quantities on each triplicate and TAR to cover several months' supply.

Fisher's patients went to the Shasta Pharmacy because other pharmacies in the Redding area refused to dispense pain medications to them. This was largely due to an ongoing fraud investigation of Dr. Fisher that was initiated by the California Attorney General's office beginning in mid-1996. Part of the investigation involved agents visiting pharmacies in area asking about Dr. Fisher's prescription practices. This frightened many pharmacists, and fearing possible repercussions, they stopped filling Dr. Fisher's prescriptions. Shasta Pharmacy was one of the few drug stores in the area that was still willing to fill Dr. Fisher's pain prescriptions. This dramatically increased the volume of pain medications that Shasta purchased and dispensed to patients.

Ironically, the AG used the increased number of TARs submitted by Shasta, resulting from its investigation, as evidence of a criminal conspiracy. For example, in 1998, Medi-Cal received between 10 and 12 TAR requests a day from Shasta to authorize payment for pain medications such as Vicodin and Soma. Rutan testified that this was comparable to the volume of TARs requested by a large medical center such as the University of California, Davis, or a large nursing or long-term care facility. It was not normal for a small retail pharmacy such as Shasta. Rutan and members of her department counted the pills that Dr. Fisher prescribed pain patients, and red flags went up when more pills were prescribed to patients in order to relieve their pain. Without examining the patients' medical records and talking to Dr. Fisher, Medi-Cal agents had no way of knowing what the level of pain was that patients were experiencing nor what level of medication was necessary to alleviate their pain.

The government referred to Dr. Fisher as "Doctor Feelgood" and repeated the earlier fraud charge that he typically spent five minutes or less with patients in the clinic and gave them prescriptions for Vicodin and Soma that were not medically necessary and that Dr. Fisher was billing for a higher level of service than he provided (i.e., up-coding).[49]

During the AG's investigation, the government sent at least seven undercover agents into Dr. Fisher's clinic wired with listening devices to gather evidence against him. Agents were instructed not to complain of any pain symptoms what would justify receiving narcotic prescriptions.

Dr. Fisher refused every request made by undercover agents. Despite the failure of investigators to fraudulently obtain narcotics from Frank Fisher, the

AG persisted in the investigation and prosecution of Dr. Fisher for eight years until a Redding jury finally acquitted him of fraud in 2004.[50]

Rutan Initiates the Prosecution

The AG's case against Dr. Fisher and the Millers was set in motion by Joyce Rutan after the meeting in Senator Greene's office. In August of 1998, she met with Harry Blair of the California Department of Justice (DOJ) at a meeting of the audit and fraud investigations committee.[51] Rutan informed Blair about the high volume of TARs for Vicodin and Soma prescriptions written by Dr. Fisher and submitted by the Shasta Pharmacy for Medi-Cal reimbursement. Blair informed Rutan that the DOJ had previously filed fraud charges against Dr. Fisher in April of 1998, and urged her to officially report her suspicions of Dr. Fisher's conspiracy and drug diversion to the DOJ.[52]

After the meeting in Senator Greene's office in October 1998, and shortly after the ALJ ruling on February 3, ordering Rutan to pay for the TARs denied by Medi-Cal, Rutan followed Blair's advice and filed a complaint with the DOJ against Dr. Fisher and the Millers. She filed a complaint on behalf of the state AG's office that formed the basis of a search warrant of Fisher's clinic and the Millers' pharmacy and their arrest.[53]

In the declaration, Rutan stated her suspicions of Fisher and the Millers' conspiracy, based simply upon the presence of Dr. Fisher and Madeline Miller, along with an attorney, at a meeting in Senator Greene's office. In court testimony, Rutan said, "In my mind, it was unusual that a physician would show up at a meeting that was supposed to discuss TAR adjudication."[54]

Rutan's declaration to the DOJ was the basis of the search warrant that the AG's office obtained to search Dr. Fisher's clinic and Shasta Pharmacy on February 18 and arrest them for alleged conspiracy. Indeed, it became the basis for count number 8, a conspiracy charge, one of 24 felony charges filed against Fisher and the Millers.

Furthermore, as a result of the arrest of Dr. Fisher and the Millers, and the seizure of patients' records, the patients whose TAR denials were scheduled to be heard April 1999 did not attend the court hearings. They knew that without the medical records and legal counsel, they could not make a case of the "medical necessity" for the medications. At the time the hearings were held, 35 Medi-Cal patients did not show up, and most of the others were postponed.

One consequence of putting Dr. Fisher and the Millers in jail without bond was that hundreds of pain patients were forced to suffer pain and withdrawal from medication without treatment or referral to other doctors. Indeed, since the AG had seized their medical records, it was virtually impossible for them to medically justify further treatment for their suffering.

The Conspiracy Charge

The government's charges against Fisher and the Millers were predicated on the claim that they were part of a "scheme" or conspiracy to create and maintain addicts in order to enrich themselves at the expense of California's Medi-Cal program. The prosecution asserted that Frank Fisher operated a "script mill" and sent addicts to the Shasta Pharmacy where the Millers supplied them with narcotics in return for kickbacks.

The problem with this was that the government produced no evidence to support the charge. In fact, the only government witness who gave testimony supporting the conspiracy charge was that of a patient named David Kupiewsky. Kupiewsky, who had suffered from seven years of self-induced, drug-related schizophrenia, was being treated for hallucinations. He was facing a six-year prison sentence for petty theft with a prior record. Under the circumstances, he agreed to be a government informer against Dr. Fisher and the Millers in return for a lenient sentence.

Kurpiewsky went into Dr. Fisher's clinic wired with a listening device to record Fisher's statement that he was involved in a conspiracy with the Shasta Pharmacy and to obtain oxycodone. The recording device malfunctioned, and he did not get a prescription for oxycodone, however. Nevertheless, the government put him on the witness stand at the trial to testify that Dr. Fisher had confided in him about a "kickback" scheme with the Millers. At the time, Kurpiewsky was experiencing hallucinations, and the presiding judge, William Gallagher, ruled that Kurpiewsky's testimony was not believable.[55]

Murder and Manslaughter Charges

Dr. Frank Fisher and the Millers were originally charged with nine counts of second-degree murder. The AG charged Dr. Fisher with the murders of his patients Rebecca Mae Williams, Tamara Lorette Stevens, and Bruce Ingomar Johannsen, Jr. To these deaths, the state later added Evelyn Nicholson and Maurina Havens. At the preliminary hearings in July 1999, Judge William D. Gallaher dismissed two of the murder charges (Williams and Stevens) on grounds of insufficient evidence.

Indeed, the prosecution's murder charges against Dr. Fisher were absurd. For example, one alleged "murder victim" Rebecca Williams died as a result of an automobile accident in which she was a passenger. Williams died as a result of massive multiple injuries, including some to her head and heart, when the car crashed into a telephone pole. The AG claimed that the pain medication that Dr. Fisher prescribed to Williams was the cause of death. They made this claim despite the fact that Rebecca Williams was alert and talking to a store salesman and paid a utility bill just before the accident.

The judge downgraded the murder charges to involuntary manslaughter in the remaining three cases (Johannsen, Nicholson, and Havens), all of whom died of drug overdoses. Stephen Miller, the pharmacist who filled Dr. Fisher's prescriptions for Nicholson and Havens, was also charged with manslaughter. Involuntary manslaughter requires proof that a human being was killed and that the killing was unlawful. A killing is unlawful if there is action that is dangerous to human life or there are "negligent acts which are aggravated, reckless, and gross" involving a high risk of death or bodily harm.[56]

The government's case was based upon the testimony of several expert witnesses that Dr. Fisher was guilty of aggravated, reckless, or gross negligence in the deaths of three patients. Two expert witnesses, Dr. Ann Murphy and Dr. David Smith, were not specialized in the treatment of CIP and thus provided highly dubious testimony about the recklessness of Dr. Fisher treatment of CIP patients. Dr. Murphy was the director of the Shasta Community Health Center and took the position that narcotic pain medication should only be given to terminal cancer patients. Indeed, there were signs at her clinic warning patients that they could not obtain opiates "no matter what their medical need or condition."[57] Dr. Smith was the well-known founder of the Haight Ashbury Free Medical Clinic in San Francisco. Smith's clinic is designed to detox a largely addict population, and therefore he avoided the use of narcotic pain medication.

Despite the expert witness testimony, the prosecution's case collapsed. For example, Bruce Johannsen, Jr., was a former patient of Dr. Fisher who was discharged from Fisher's care two months before his death and who bought the narcotics that killed him illegally off the street, not from Frank Fisher.

Evelyn Nicholson suffered from serious back pain, going to the emergency room of the hospital 10-12 times the previous year. She suffered from manic depression and had made multiple suicide attempts. In addition to taking her pain medication as prescribed by Dr. Fisher, she was drinking alcohol the night before her death as well as taking cough syrup with codeine. She died in her bed from an unintentional overdose of multiple drugs or suicide. Maurina Havens also died from an overdose of multiple drugs on March 3, 1999, almost three weeks after Dr. Fisher was arrested. Her husband reported that she became deeply depressed after Dr. Fisher's arrest and took her own life.

The only government expert witness with experience treating CIP, Dr. Eisele, testified that he "saw nothing in the files to indicate that Dr. Fisher was not practicing in good faith."[58] The charges of manslaughter were clearly ludicrous, and the judge dismissed them as he had done previously with the murder charges.

Disruption of Dr. Fisher's and the Millers' Lives

Despite the exoneration of Frank Fisher and the Millers, the ordeal has destroyed their lives and careers and that of hundreds of their patients. The government seized Dr. Fisher's clinic, which had a dozen employees and a gross income of about a million dollars. His personal assets amounting to $50,000 was also seized. His aging parents depleted their retirement savings by $100,000 for their son's legal defense. At 50 years of age, he was forced to move back into his parents' home, living in his childhood room for the past five and a half years. He drove a 1988 Mercedez with about 300,000 miles on it.

Madeline and Steven Miller were likewise devastated by the prosecution. Their pharmacy and assets amounting to about $400,000 in value were seized, and the government sought to revoke Steven Miller's pharmacy license. While they were in jail and did not have access to their financial resources, they were unable to make their mortgage payments on their home and thus lost it.

9

DEA SHOW TRIAL: "MAGICAL MOMENTS" OF THE COMPREHENSIVE CARE CONSPIRACY

The Drug Enforcement Agency's (DEA) Comprehensive Care case in Myrtle Beach, South Carolina, in 2002 was its biggest criminal case against nine doctors charged with overprescribing narcotics. The prosecutor, assistant U.S. Attorney Bill Day, said, "If doctors have a doubt whether they could get in trouble, this case should answer that."[1] Comprehensive Care illustrates the enormous pressure that the DEA can place upon physicians to testify falsely against other doctors. It also illustrates the nature of a state medical board's role in working with the DEA in prosecuting physicians.[2]

On June 25, 2002, nine doctors and three employees of the Myrtle Beach Comprehensive Care and Pain Management Center (Comprehensive Care), a pain clinic, were indicted by the Federal government on 93 counts of illegal activity at the clinic between 1997 and 2001. The charges included conspiracy to distribute narcotics, laundering money, and health care billing fraud.

The DEA threatened Dr. David Michael Woodward, the owner and executive director of the clinic, with 60 years in prison, the incarceration of his wife who was a part-time employee, and seizure of all of his assets. If the Woodwards were convicted, it would have resulted in the abandonment of their two young children, one of whom had incurable cystic fibrosis. Woodward feared that his children would be left without financial support and critically needed health insurance.

Hoping for leniency, Woodward agreed to plead guilty to all of the DEA's charges on January 7, 2003, and testify against the doctors who worked for him during five years at the clinic.[3] He testified that they were all part of an illegal conspiracy to distribute narcotics, commit Medicare and Medicaid fraud, and launder the illegal money by putting it back into his business. In exchange for the testimony, the DEA offered Woodward a plea agreement, verbally promising him two or three years in jail, not indicting his wife, and allowing him to keep up to half of his assets.

Woodward's testimony against the doctors set off a panic among them. Fearing the destruction of their families and facing life in prison, five of the doctors pled guilty and agreed to testify against their colleagues at trial. One physician, Benjamin Moore, agreed to plead guilty but later in a pang of conscience, committed suicide rather than testify against his colleagues.[4] Three doctors, Michael Jackson, 55, Ricardo Alerre, 73, and Deborah Bordeaux, 50, refused to plead guilty to the charges and instead went to trial.

A "WELL-RESPECTED" NEUROLOGIST

Dr. Michael Woodward was uniquely qualified for the newly emerging field of pain management. He graduated from the University of Georgia with a degree in biochemistry and microbiology in 1981 and then earned a combined master's degree in business administration and a law degree in 1986 from the University of Georgia. Woodward received his medical degree from Mercer University School of Medicine in 1989, and undertook a three-year residency training in neurology (diseases of the brain, spinal chord, and peripheral nerves) at Yale University School of Medicine. He also undertook a two-year master's degree program in health care administration at the University of Florida in 2001.

Woodward finished his medical training in 1993 and moved to Myrtle Beach, South Carolina, where he opened up a solo practice in Neurology and Sleep Disorders Medicine. A year later, he purchased a building for his clinic in Myrtle Beach and changed the name of the practice to Comprehensive Care and Pain Management Center. The pain center continued to operate until it was closed by the DEA in 2001.

In 1996, Woodward passed his board exams in pain management, which is administered by the nationally recognized American Academy of Pain Management. Pain management is a subspecialty of neurology. Woodward decided to go into this specialty because there was a great demand for it in South Carolina. Indeed, Woodward estimated that 95 percent of his clinic work was in pain management.

This is not surprising given the fact that, in 2001, there were only 10 pain specialists in all of South Carolina, which has a population of 4.1 million. There was one pain doctor in Columbia, two in Greenville, one in Hilton Head, one in Lexington, one in Mt. Pleasant, two in Myrtle Beach, and two in Spartanburg.[5] Given the scarcity of pain specialists in the state, patients were forced to travel long distances to Comprehensive Care for treatment.

WOODWARD'S LEGAL BATTLE WITH THE MEDICAL BOARD

Dr. Woodward had a long-running legal battle with the South Carolina State Board of Medicine, supported by the DEA from the beginning of his practice.[6] Dr. Ben C. Pendarvis, Jr., and Dr. Hartwell Z. Hildebrand served on the medical board from 1993 to 2000 as president and vice president of the board. Dr. Hildebrand played a critical role in gathering information for the complaint against Dr. Woodward and as vice president of the board, he chaired the meeting at which the decision was made to suspend Woodward's medical license. The DEA took its cues from the board and carried out a five-year investigation of Woodward's clinic including three raids of the clinic in 1996, 1998, and in June 2000 before it finally closed Comprehensive Care in June 2001. The raids in 1996, 1998, and 2000 apparently did not provide evidence of any criminal wrongdoing, but that did not deter the DEA.

Hildebrand and members of the board believed that opioids should be used primarily for end-of-life treatment. They viewed tolerance and dependence as addiction and the use of opioids as masking the underlying cause of pain. In prosecuting Dr. Woodward, the DEA had all the board's disciplinary documentation. All it had to do is elaborate upon the board's position concerning Dr. Woodward. For example, in 1966, the board charged Woodward with "giving controlled substances (to 12 patients) without valid medical justification."[7] This was repeated in board documents issued from 1996 to 2000. In 2000, Linda Traub, a diversion officer, took the board's cue when she told Dr. Benjamin Moore that "opiates were only for terminal cancer patients" and warned him not to prescribe Oxycontin.[8]

In 1995, the board first reprimanded Woodward based upon a minor complaint that from 1993 to 1994, he refused to provide copies of three patient's medical records to the board. The board fined him $3,000, ordered him to provide records to his patients, and take a Quality Medical Recordkeeping course for Health Care Professionals administered by the Florida Medical Association.

Woodward regarded the clinic's patient records as his property and resented the board's meddling, so he dragged his feet in responding to the board's reprimand. He partially complied with the order by paying the fine in October 1995, and gave the three patients their medical records. He did not provide proof of having taken the recordkeeping course, however. The board responded by suspending his medical license on November 12. He subsequently provided the necessary proof of completing the course, and his license was reinstated on November 15.

On December 4, 1996, the board again filed charges against Dr. Woodward. This was based upon an investigation carried out by Dr. Hildebrand, the board vice president, and Dr. Stephen Schabel (a former board member), who were on the board's disciplinary Investigative Review Committee (IRC). The IRC met on October 10, 1996, and made a recommendation to the medical board to suspend Woodward's medical license.

Dr. Hildebrand was involved in gathering documentation from patients who complained about Woodward. The board concluded that Woodward was guilty of unethical sexual conduct with two female patients, overprescribing Stadol to patients without medical justification, and committing fraud by testing unnecessarily. These charges later formed the basis of the DEA's indictment against Dr. Woodward and of all the doctors who worked at the clinic. The principal difference between the board's charges and the DEA's was that instead of Stadol, the DEA charged the doctors with overprescribing OxyContin. OxyContin was not widely available in 1996, and the criminal penalties for OxyContin were much greater than for Stadol.

Dr. Woodward asked the board to subpoena the patients who filed complaints against him in order to challenge their credibility. He had documents that focused on one of them, a former employee, was addicted to Stadol and illegally called in prescriptions for herself using patients' names. He also wanted the board to adopt a pain management guideline following the Federation of State Medical Boards in order to justify his prescription of Stadol to relieve chronic pain. Indeed, the board did not adopt pain management guidelines until February 1999. Woodward has taken credit for the board's decision to adopt treatment pain guidelines.

Woodward also challenged the board's expert witnesses on the grounds that they were not pain or sleep study specialists, and he submitted affidavits from pain management experts attesting to the legitimacy of his use of Stadol for pain patients. There was even expert testimony that the female patients who claimed Dr. Woodward sexually molested them may have been hallucinating from the use of Stadol.[9]

The board rejected most of Woodward's requests and decided to suspend his medical license on October 21, 1997. They gave three reasons for this action:

1. Dr. Woodward had sexual conduct with two patients that was unethical and unprofessional.
2. Woodward overprescribed controlled substances—mostly Stadol—to 12 patients without valid medical justification.
3. He kept inadequate patient records for patients' diagnosis, assessment and treatment, including monitoring the effects of drugs.

The DEA followed the lead of the board and also suspended Woodward's license to prescribe controlled substances. Woodward appealed the board's decision to an administrative law judge who reinstated his medical license two months later in December 1997. The judge ruled that Dr. Hildebrand and the board carried out a "one-sided investigation" of Woodward and violated the South Carolina constitution, which demands separation of prosecutorial and adjudicative functions of professional regulatory boards. By chairing the IRC that investigated Woodward and also participating in the board meeting that suspended his license, Dr. Hildebrand had violated Woodward's constitutional rights. The judge said that the board had been motivated by a "will-to-win."[10]

Despite this sharp rebuke of the medical board, it remained intransigent and met on July 22, 1998 to revoke his license again. Woodward appealed the decision to the administrative law judge and then to the Fifth Judicial Circuit court, and in March 2000, he succeeded in overturning the action of the board and having his medical license reinstated. The board stubbornly refused to give in and immediately appealed the reinstatement of Woodward's license. The issue was still pending at the time that the DEA intervened to close the clinic in 2001.

A New Business Model

The suspensions of Dr. Woodward's medical and DEA licenses created severe staffing problems at the clinic. He was forced to hire "proxy" physicians to keep the clinic open. Woodward testified that in December 1996, for example, he became aware that he might lose his medical license. In anticipation, he began to look for a doctor to replace him.[11]

After he lost his license in 1997, Woodward was forced to use a *locum tenens* "rent-a-doc" company called Med Pro based in Atlanta, Georgia, to staff his practice. Indeed, during the periods in which he had a medical but not a DEA license, he adopted a procedure he called training or "shadowing." He instructed *locum tenens* doctors to accompany him while examining patients and asked them to sign prescriptions for the patients.

In order to comply with the medical board's reprimand, Woodward insisted that all patients needed a current Magnetic Resonance Imaging and Nerve Conduction Study on file. If they did not have one, they were given three months to get it or they were terminated. Never mind the fact that no magnetic resonance imaging, electromyogram, or nerve conduction study will ever rule in or out whether a patient has chronic pain.

Patient charts were to be computer-generated so that even if a doctor neglected some component of the patient's history, physical, diagnosis, or treatment, the computer would automatically add information about the patient from the previous visit. This was used by the prosecution in the trial as evidence of a conspiracy. The same wording on all patient charts was described by prosecutors as scamming with the intent to defraud.

Ironically, Dr. Woodward's efforts to comply with the medical board's demands were used against him and all the doctors who worked for him at the clinic. For example, when Woodward lost his medical license, there was no one in the clinic qualified to read the electroencephalogram sleep tests. When he got his license back, he resumed reading them, but there was an eight-month delay in adding the test results to the patient's chart. Since the clinic had already billed for the procedure but it was not yet entered into the patient's chart, the DEA interpreted this as evidence of fraud and claimed the tests were never performed.

Likewise, what the prosecution called "fast-tracking" patients was also connected with the staffing problems at the clinic. This was the practice of a doctor seeing several patients all together. Often, it was just a matter of writing a prescription that the patient was already on and had no medical complaints. During the trial, Dr. Michael Jackson explained that "fast-tracking" was not illegal and was a common practice in the military and largest hospitals in the United States. Nevertheless, Dr. Woodward opposed fast-tracking, and it occurred only when there was a severe staff shortage and Woodward was not around.[12]

According to Dr. Gregory W. Walter, a physician who worked at Comprehensive Care, after the DEA raids keeping the clinic open was like a "Chinese fire drill." All sorts of employees at the clinic were quitting on a daily basis. There were between 60 and 80 patients a day, most of whom were returning for prescription refills. The waiting room of the clinic was described as a "bad motorcycle rally" with no children and lots of people with tattoos and piercing.[13] When Woodward had only one doctor on staff, he was pushed to the limit all day long. This meant that he had to adopt short cuts to see the patients. When he had two doctors on staff at the clinic, such as Drs. Alerre and Moore, Woodward used their DEA certificates to prescribe medications to patients.

Walter has questioned the DEA's conspiracy charges in the following way.[14] He knew of no conspiracy by the doctors at Comprehensive Care to commit fraud. Indeed, Dr. Walter and other *locum tenens* doctors were paid a flat rate of about $20 per patient, and they received nothing for writing prescriptions.

Woodward himself did not believe that he had committed fraud until after he was indicted and sent to prison. Indeed, at the trial, Woodward testified that it was only after he pled guilty and was in prison that he came to recognize that his practice constituted a conspiracy. He said, "Upon reviewing the materials in the case, I came to the conclusion" I was guilty.[15]

Billing Fraud

All of the billing occurred upstairs in the manager's office. The physicians were not involved in billing at the clinic and almost never went upstairs to the office. Likewise, on advice from his attorney, Woodward did not go downstairs where the physicians examined patients during the periods that his medical license was suspended. He spent much of his time in the office with the billing manager, Pamela Wagner. The assumption by the staff was that Woodward and Wagner were romantically linked.

David Von Vandergriff, a Ph.D. in educational counseling, started working at Comprehensive Care in October 1998. In October 1999, he was promoted to executive director, managing the clinic. In January 2000, Vandergriff was fired by Woodward because he allowed the doctors to practice fast-tracking. Vandergriff claimed that Woodward had not fired him, but decided to leave Comprehensive Care because Woodward was manic-depressive and his moods swung wildly from a calm demeanor to hostile and aggressive behavior.

Vandergriff was arrested in 1999 and pled guilty to defrauding his former employer, the Marion-Dillon county Board of Disability and Special Needs. After leaving Comprehensive Care in 2000, he also pled guilty to fraudulently billing at the clinic. Wendy Suggs, the office manager, and her son Tim also pled guilty to fraudulent billing in concert with Vandergriff. For example, Vandergriff hired Wendy Suggs' son, Tim, to do the nerve conduction studies at the clinic. However, Tim Suggs was not licensed to do the studies and his equipment was not even properly calibrated to work. Hence, the results of the tests were falsified.[16]

After leaving Comprehensive Care, Vandergriff established a rival pain clinic in Myrtle Beach with doctors who were formerly employed at Comprehensive Care. Before he established the rival clinic, however, he contacted the DEA, offering to provide information about Woodward's fraudulent billing practices at Comprehensive Care. He also arranged to have the doctors at his new clinic testify against Woodward. He did this in hope of making a deal to mitigate the charges against him for stealing money from the handicapped children's program for which he was arrested in 1999 and committing fraud at Comprehensive Care. He was successful insofar as he received only 12 months in prison for both crimes.[17]

Unsuspecting *Locum Tenens* Doctors

Comprehensive Care was under criminal investigation by the DEA since 1996. And yet eight doctors were allowed to join the practice over the next five years without any caution or warning from the authorities. Since the DEA had to approve any change in a doctor's address, it implicitly gave them its blessing to work at the clinic.

Contrary to the DEA's charge that the doctors at Comprehensive Care were part of a criminal conspiracy, they were all misled by the *locum tenens* recruiting companies. It would have been virtually impossible for the doctors to have conspired to do what they were accused of doing when they were recruited by a short-term *locum tenens* company. They arrived at different times from different parts of the country, they did not know one another beforehand, and most of them stayed less than one year. Dr. Deborah Bordeaux, for example, worked at the clinic for only 55 days.

The South Carolina Medical Board and the DEA also misled the doctors into believing that Comprehensive Care was a legitimate medical practice. All the physicians believed that Michael Woodward had an outstanding professional reputation.

Dr. Ben Moore's recruiting experience illustrates this. From June 1999 to May 2000, just before being hired by Woodward, he worked at three different family practice clinics with excellent references from each. Unfortunately, they all went bankrupt, and he had to move three times during that period to find employment—the third time from California to North Carolina. His last employer, Onslow County Hospital in North Carolina, decided to sell off the clinic in 2000; thus Dr. Moore was once again unemployed. As an independent contractor, he had no unemployment insurance and no savings. He was eager to find employment. Just as he was about to leave a motel in North Carolina to return to California, he was paged by Med-Pro. It told him about a job at a "chronic pain clinic" in Myrtle Beach, South Carolina. The recruiter said that the owner was a "well-respected" neurologist who was "certified" in pain management and that his employees recently walked out on him to start their own clinic. Ben Moore thought that this was typical bickering between doctors and thought nothing more about it.

In fact, Moore was highly impressed by Woodward's medical credentials. He was a Yale-trained doctor in neurology and was a chief resident. Woodward was Board Certified by the American Academy of Pain Management. Moore even called the South Carolina Board of Medical Examiners to check out Woodward's professional reputation and was told that "Dr. Woodward had a full and unlimited license to practice medicine."[18] They faxed him the South Carolina Medical Board Guidelines on the use of controlled substances but did not mention the fact that the board had suspended Woodward's license three times and was currently appealing the Fifth Circuit Court's decision to reinstate his license.

Ben Moore compared the medical board's guidelines for prescribing opioids with Woodward's protocol at Comprehensive Care[19] and with the University of North Carolina at Chapel Hill, where he had completed a two-year residency from 1991–1993 in neurology, including training at the University of North Carolina Pain Clinic.[20] All three of the guidelines were consistent and state-of-the-art. In addition, Moore was reassured by a speech given by Pat Good, the Chief of Liaison and Policy at the Diversion Division of DEA in 1998. Good said that "a physician need not fear DEA action of prescribing controlled substances in good faith for legitimate medical purpose."[21]

When Moore asked Woodward about the three doctors who left the clinic *en masse*, he was misleadingly told that he fired them because they illegally engaged in "fast-tracking" patients during his absence from the clinic. Drs. Alerre and Bordeaux had never seen more than one patient at a time, and Drs. Jackson, Sutherland, and Bordeaux quit Comprehensive Care; they were not fired.

On June 13, 2000, only 19 days after Moore started working at the clinic, the DEA carried out its third raid of the clinic seizing patient files, records, and downloading computer files. Agent Traub told Moore he was not under investigation and that nothing he said to her would be held against him. She told him not to use OxyContin but never told him to leave the practice. The DEA failed to find evidence of fraud or diversion, however. Rather than cease its criminal investigation, the DEA redoubled its efforts to find evidence of criminal wrongdoing.

Moore resigned after the raid and for the next three weeks tried to find another job, without success. He contacted the recruiting agency, Med Pro, and told it what had happened and said he was not happy at Comprehensive Care and would like to find alternative employment. There was nothing available at the time. Woodward persuaded him to stay by explaining that the DEA raid was connected to the "fast-tracking" doctors who were no longer at the clinic. Moore naively accepted this explanation and decided to continue working at the clinic until he was able to find another job. What he did not realize was that because of the DEA raids on Comprehensive Care, no other clinic or hospital would hire him.

In early 2000, the DEA forced four more doctors out of the clinic for having their previous place of employment on their DEA registration. In other words, instead of simply updating their new employment address, it informed the doctors that they were not authorized to work at Comprehensive Care. When the doctors resigned, it left hundreds of patients with no help to wean them off their medication and no pain specialist to continue their therapy. Moore was the last doctor left in the clinic, and the DEA suspended his license in 2001 in order to close the clinic.

"Magical Moments" of Conspiracy

During the trial, the prosecution used a novel and fantastical conspiracy theory to convict Drs. Jackson, Alerre, and Bordeaux. David Woodward was the star witness against the doctors. Indeed, the U.S. Court of Appeals ruled in 2005 that Dr. Woodward's testimony alone was sufficient to convict the doctors.[22] The basis of Woodward's conspiracy claim was that he had "magical moments" with all three of the doctors.

Woodward incredulously testified that he had experienced "magical moments" of conspiracy awareness with the doctors.[23] He said that at these moments he knew the doctors were "part of his (criminal) team."[24] In the case of Michael Jackson who was hired in 1998, Woodward asked, "Are you going to be able to do this?" Dr. Jackson reportedly responded, "I got your back." Woodward interpreted this remark to mean Jackson understood that he was part of the conspiracy.[25]

Woodward allegedly asked Dr. Alerre if he was comfortable with "what we were doing." Alerre said "Oh, to hell with it."[26] Woodward said that he understood Alerre's remarks as confirmation that he was "part of our team," that is, Woodward's illegal conspiracy.

In the case of Dr. Bordeaux, Woodward allegedly asked her if she "understood what we're doing and all that?"[27] She reportedly replied that she was having car and financial troubles and responded, "If I go along with this, can I have your father's pickup truck?"

Woodward's Implausible Testimony

The accused doctors' accounts of the referenced conversations with Woodward are at great variance. For example, Dr. Jackson recounted a conversation with Woodward that bore some resemblance to a conversion that occurred after Dr. Jackson was recruited in April 1998. Jackson was being trained by Woodward to treat chronic pain patients. At that time, Dr. Woodward told Jackson that he may lose his license and that was why he spent extra time training him. Woodward asked Jackson if he knew what he was doing, and Jackson replied yes. Woodward then reminded Jackson that he may lose his license and at that point Dr. Jackson said, "I've got your back."[28] This comment had nothing to do with a criminal conspiracy, but was rather Jackson's expression of support for Woodward in the event he lost his medical license.

During cross-examination Dr. Alerre was asked about Woodward's magical moment or "bright line of conspiracy." Alerre's response was that the term "magical moment" was a "ridiculous expression." When he was asked if he was "getting paid to be in an illegal pill mill," he said, "I'm too old to think about that." When Alerre was directly asked about Woodward's reported conversation he said that "if he said that, I wouldn't say I'll kill him, but no, he didn't."[29] Dr. Alerre was 73 years old, a retired lieutenant colonel Air Force surgeon and was working part-time at the clinic.

The most imaginative claim about conspiracy concerned Woodward's assertion about an alleged conversation with Dr. Bordeaux. Woodward testified that Bordeaux was having a hard time financially and had car trouble.[30] She reportedly asked to have Woodward's old pickup truck. This claim is without any factual foundation. During her brief employment at Comprehensive Care, Dr. Bordeaux had several cars registered in her name that were in excellent working condition. She had a 1995 Chevrolet Lumina in perfect mechanical condition, a 1997 GMC pick-up and her son had a restored 1967 Mustang in showroom condition. He also had a 1989 Toyota Celica that was also mechanically sound. The only reference she ever made to Woodward about his father's old, rusted-out pick-up truck was to ask if he would move it from clinic's parking lot so she could park there.

Dr. Bordeaux's court-appointed attorney failed to challenge Woodward's incredulous "magical moments" testimony. Indeed, she tried without success to get a new attorney to represent her. Bordeaux claimed her attorney, R. Scott Joye, was grossly negligent. For example, at a meeting requested by William Day, the assistant U.S. Attorney prosecuting the case, her attorney, R. Scott Joye, acknowledged that he had not yet read the files Dr. Bordeaux had given him and said almost nothing at the meeting.[31]

Joye subsequently went on a three-week vacation in Mexico, despite the fact that the trial was set to begin on September 16, 2002. He repeatedly pressured Bordeaux to plea-bargain with the DEA using the colorful expression "the fist pig to the trough gets the best food, and the first person to make a deal will get the best deal." Finally, Joye also had a potential conflict of interest insofar as he represented a notorious biker bar in Horry County, which reportedly was under investigation for illegal drugs by the DEA and U.S. Attorney—the very agencies prosecuting his client, Dr. Bordeaux.

Outcome of the Case

The DEA's prosecution of the Comprehensive Care case resulted in its biggest success involving doctors charged with overprescribing narcotics. The federal investigation resulted in a total of 27 convictions, including 8 former clinic doctors and 1 doctor who committed suicide before trial.

The success of their case was based largely upon the self-serving testimony of the owner of a pain clinic, Dr. Michael Woodward. He testified against all of his employees for a reduced sentence. Ironically, instead of the two to three years he was promised by the DEA, Woodward received 15 years in prison and lost his entire assets. He has been held in solitary confinement since he was arrested in 2002 and is let out only to testify against other doctors who are prosecuted by the DEA throughout the country.

Five *locum tenens* doctors at Comprehensive Care received prison sentences of between two and three years, lost their licenses to practice medicine, and their assets. Of the three doctors who went to trial, Dr. Michael D. Jackson received a prison sentence of 24 years, Dr. Deborah Bordeaux 19 years, and Dr. Ricardo Alerre 8 years.[32] Thus the South Carolina Medical Board, working in concert with the DEA, used Woodward's testimony to destroy the careers and lives of nine dedicated doctors, including the suicide death of a devoted and honorable physician, Benjamin Moore. It also left hundreds of patients in chronic pain with no place to receive medical treatment. Nevertheless, the DEA holds up Comprehensive Care as a highly successful model of illegal drug prosecution.

10

CONCLUSION

The government has made medical doctors scapegoats for the financial crisis of health care in the country and for the failed war on drugs. Physicians' role as sacrificial lambs follows the long history of political scapegoats in the United States. Beginning with the Salem witch trials, the lynching of blacks during the civil war and the depression of the 1930s, the Japanese reconcentration camps, and communist scapegoats of the McCarthy era, the government has blamed specific groups for societal turmoil and instability.

Physicians have become the enemies of the country's health care. This is comparable to the anti-Communist spy investigations of the 1950s. The government has declared that doctors and other health professionals constitute a threat to the nation's health. Comparable to the blacklist, the lives of many innocent physicians have been destroyed by criminal investigations, fines, and criminal prosecutions.

The book has documented the government's draconian policy of prosecuting physicians for medical fraud, kickbacks, and drug diversion. It contains numerous cases of doctors who were tried for criminal felonies for making innocent billing mistakes or naively accepting directorships of clinics. They lost all of their savings and assets, received prison sentences, and some have been driven to suicide rather than live with the disgrace to their families. Physicians who have been scammed by drug addicts or dealers into giving them pain medicine have also lost everything and some have been given life sentences in prison. Their families have been destroyed in the process, and thousands of patients have been left without their medical care.

Political scapegoating is particularly evident during periods of social and economic instability whenever there is a failure to meet societal expectations. The widespread fear that the government cannot pay for the out-of-control costs of Medicare and the explosive costs of heath services has fed societal anxiety. Likewise, the failure of the war on drugs has made doctors an ideal scapegoat for a new drug epidemic—prescription painkillers.

The physician as scapegoat is important to politicians both to blame for a major threat to society and it promises a relatively easy and inexpensive solution. The solution is to eliminate wealthy and corrupt doctors who threaten the nation's health care. A tough law and order campaign against corrupt doctors therefore creates the illusion that the state is acting as the protector of the citizenry.

Scapegoats and villains have been blamed for a wide variety of social ills in society from unemployment and crime to threats to national security. Scapegoats are the inverse of societal heroes. They are widely perceived to be guilty and are subject to stated and implied accusations of wrongdoing. They are also subject to public ridicule and investigations.

This stands in stark contrast with the former hero image of doctors symbolized by the late Surgeon General C. Everett Koop who was widely held to be moral, competent, and selfless. Since the 1980s, doctors have suffered an image collapse and are now viewed as arrogant, corrupt, and above the law. Many are seen primarily as entrepreneurs enriching themselves at the expense of senior citizens and the roughly 46 million citizens who lack health insurance.

Medical doctors fit the pattern of a group suffering from a collapse of their image. They do not recognize that there is a national political campaign against them for fraud, kickbacks, and drug diversion. Instead, they see themselves as victims of local vendettas by ambitious prosecutors, competitors, and troubled or greedy whistleblowers. Like other scapegoats, they tend believe that their cases are individual and unique to them. This explains the fact that physicians turn their backs on other doctors who have been egregiously targeted by the government for investigation and prosecution.

Scapegoats do not see the broader aspects of their collapsed credibility. Societal scapegoats are deemed to have violated a code of conduct. A scapegoat is already found guilty before he is indicted or tried; there is widespread societal consensus that what he did was wrong. This is reflected in trials of physicians where judges and juries dismiss most of the charges against doctors but invariably convict them of some wrongdoing. The prevailing consensus is that they must be guilty of something or why else would the government bring charges against them.

The history of scapegoats is that once they have been stigmatized, they will continue to be abused by the government in the future. The only way to transform a scapegoats' public image is to first recognize that they are political scapegoats. This has occurred twice. The first time was during the 1920s when doctors were made scapegoats in the first war on drugs. It happened again in 1990, when medical associations throughout the United States supported a call by the American Medical Association (AMA) for the resignation of the Inspector General of the HHS for his role in Medicare/Medicaid fraud investigation abuses targeting doctors.

In both instances, the leadership of the AMA called a halt to the senseless destruction of doctors' careers and lives in the government's vain pursuit of drug addicts who were treated by physicians and to stamp-out medical fraud. The president of the AMA contacted the president of the United States in both cases and demanded an end to the witch hunts.

Similarly, in order to end the government's current war on doctors it will be necessary for medical associations to launch a national campaign to demand an end to the unjust prosecution of physicians.

Notes

Chapter 1

1. CBS News, "U.S. Heading for Financial Trouble?," March 4, 2007, www.cbsnews.com/stories/2007/03/01/60minutes/printable252. David Walker claims that without fundamental change, the government will not have enough money for national defense, homeland security, education, or anything else.

2. Ibid.

3. Ibid. Walker points out that beginning in 2008 and for the next 20 years, 78 million American will become medical dependents of the U.S. taxpayer. When the baby boomers start retiring en mass, it will be a tsunami of spending that could swamp the ship of state.

4. Drug Policy Alliance, "Congressman Souder Afraid of Open Debate on Failed War on Drugs," February 9, 2006.

5. There is a long tradition of politicians using scapegoats to blame for social and economic illness in society. For example, the slums, corruption, and lawlessness in the big cities of American during the 1890s were blamed on immigrants. The immigrant was demonized as lawless and violent posing a threat of anarchist terror to America. The adoption of the Immigration Act of 1903 empowered the government to deport aliens simply because their presence was perceived to be a threat to the public welfare (William Preston, Jr., *Aliens and Dissenters: Federal Suppression of Radicals, 1903–1933* [Cambridge, MA: Harvard University Press], 11–34), 1966. Hollywood figures, intellectuals, and federal officials were made scapegoats during the 1940s by the House Committee on Un-American Activities and Senator Joseph McCarthy to blame for the stalemate in Korea and communist gains in the world. There is also a long history of scapegoating groups in society in the war on drugs. They included Chinese immigrants who were blamed for an opium epidemic during the 1900s, African-Americans for a cocaine epidemic during the 1930s and then again in the 1980s for a crack cocaine epidemic, Mexicans for a marijuana epidemic during the 1940s, Hippies for LSD, Marijuana and Heroin during the 1960s and doctors and pharmacists for the most recent drug war against OxyContin.

6. According to the Office of National Drug Control Policy Executive Office of the President, an emerging new drug threat is prescription drugs. Next to marijuana, OxyContin and Vicodin are the most commonly abused drugs by teens. ONDCP, "Teens

and Prescription Drugs: An Analysis of Recent Trends on the Emerging Drug Threat," February 2007, 1, 6. The DEA has identified prescription drugs as a top priority in the war on drugs. "Prescription Drug Abuse: What Is Being Done to Address This New Drug Epidemic?" Statement of Joseph T. Rannazzisi, deputy assistant administrator, Office of Diversion Control DEA, U.S. Department of Justice before the House Government Reform Committee, Subcommittee on Criminal Justice, Drug Policy and Human Resources, July 26, 2006, http://www.dea.gov/pubs/cngrtest/ct072606.html. "Doctor shopping" by drug addicts and improper prescribing by doctors are said to be the most common sources of illegal prescription drugs.

7. Malcolm K. Sparrow, *License to Steal: How Fraud Bleeds America's Health Care System* (Boulder, CO: Westview Press, 2000), viii.

8. Ibid., xvi–xvii.

9. PricewaterhouseCoopers' Health Research Institute, "Top Seven Health Industry Trends in '07," 2007, 2.

10. PriceWaterhouseCoopers, "The Factors Fueling Rising Healthcare Costs 2006," 2006, 6–8.

11. Reprinted with permission © 2006 Atlantic Information Services, Inc. Originally published in "The AIS Report on Blue Cross and Blue Shield Plans," November 2006 issue. Originally published in the April 26, 2006, issue of *Managed Care Week*.

12. CNNMoney.com, Fortune Global 500, "Industry: Health Care: Insurance & Managed Care," July 24, 2006, issue, http://Money.cnn.com/magazines/fortune/global500/2006/industries/Health_Care_Insurance_Managed_Care/1.html.

13. Ronald T. Libby, "Treating Doctors as Drug Dealers: The DEA's War on Prescription Painkillers," *Policy Analysis*, no. 545, June 16, 2005.

CHAPTER 2

1. Allen H. Moore, *Mustard Plasters and Printer's Ink* (New York: Exposition Press, 1959).

2. Ibid., 243.

3. Ibid., 105.

4. Ibid., 255–256.

5. Unbeknownst to Dr. Moore, the South Carolina Medical Board had twice revoked Dr. Woodward's medical license in 1997 and 1998 on grounds of "professional misconduct" for sexual misconduct and overprescribing drugs. Both times, Woodward's license was reinstated on the grounds of procedural irregularities. In 2001, Woodward and the board reached an agreement in which the board would dismiss the complaints and, in return, he would not apply for a license to practice in South Carolina. When Dr. Moore was hired, there were no civil or criminal charges against Woodward.

6. The Federation of State Medical Boards of the United States, Inc., "Model Guidelines for the Use of Controlled Substances for the Treatment of Pain," May 2, 1998, http://www.medsch.wisc.edu/painpolicy/domestic/model.html.

7. Letter from Dr. Benjamin R. Moore to Congressman Henry E. Brown, Jr., June 12, 2001.

8. Letter from Dr. Benjamin Moore to Congressman Mark Sanford, June 15, 2000.

9. Ibid.

10. The common strategy used by physicians for treating pain with opioid (the contemporary term for narcotics) analgesics is to provide "as-needed" intermittent

dosing with a short half-life drug (e.g., hydrocodone, hydromorphone, and codeine). However, these drugs must be taken every three to four hours, which produces anxiety and pain in patients, making it impossible to sleep through the night. By contrast, long-acting sustained-released opiods such as oxycodone, morphone, and fentanyl control pain for periods from 8 to 12 hours and as long as 72 hours.

11. Letter from Benjamin R. Moore, D.O., to the Honorable Henry Hyde, July 31, 2001.

12. The National Foundation for the Treatment of Pain, "Perspectives in Intractable Pain Management: An Analysis of Current Diverging Viewpoints," September 1, 2001, www.paincare.org.

13. Elaine Gaston, "Accused MB Doctor Yields License," *Sun News* (SC), November 15, 2001. In deciding which doctors to investigate, the DEA relies upon medication categories established in 1970 by the Controlled Substances Act. The DEA groups drugs into five different "schedules" from I to V depending upon their potential for addiction. Schedule I drugs are banned. They include marijuana, LSD, heroin, and cocaine. Schedule II are prescribed drugs and include powerful painkillers such as morphine, Dilaudid, and OxyContin. Schedule III drugs are also prescribed but include less potent drugs such as anabolic steroids, some barbiturates, and blends of aspirin and codeine. Schedule IV drugs also require prescription and include benzodiazepines such as Valium. Schedule V drugs contain some prescription drugs as well as over-the-counter cough medicines that are not addictive.

14. Kaushik Sandeep, "Anatomy of a Drug Scare," *B. Phoenix*, June 21–28, 2001. 32. Page 33.

15. Ibid.

16. Daniel Forbes, "Prime-Time Propaganda: How the White House Secretly Hood-winked Network TV on Its Anti-Drug Message," January 13, 2001. Salon.com, www.salon.com/news/feature/2000/01/13/drugs/index.htm.

17. Ibid.

18. Karin Kischer, "Congress Pushes OxyContin Fight," *Charleston Daily Mail* (West Virginia), November 19, 2001.

19. Kaushik, "Anatomy of a Drug Scare," 3.

20. Rick Bay, "The War on Drugs—A War on Sick People and Doctors," *Alternatives for Cultural Creativity*, 15 (Fall 2000), www.alternatives magazine.com.

21. In 1976, there were only 3 or 4 million heroin users in the United States. A survey conducted by the government's NIDA National Household Survey of Drug Abuse in 1987, found that very few cocaine users become addicted. Heroin use in the United States is also rare. According to the government's data, 0.2 percent of the population are users. See Jacob Sullum, *Saying Yes: In Defense of Drug Use* (New York: Jeremy P. Tarcher/Putnam, 2003), 227. Likewise, only 300,000 people used cocaine daily or nearly every day in 1988, out of 244,498,982 which is 1.2 percent of the total population. Stanton Peele, "Addiction as a Cultural Concept," *Annals of the New York Academy of Sciences*, 602(11) (1990).

22. For a discussion of the failed war on drugs, see Mike Gray, *Drug Crazy* (New York: Routledge, 2000) and David F. Musto, *The American Disease: Origins of Narcotic Control*, 3rd ed. (New York: Oxford University Press, 1999).

23. Ronald T. Libby, "Treating Doctors as Drug Dealers: The DEA's War on Pre-scription Painkillers," *Policy Analysis*, no. 545, June 16, 2005, CATO Institute, Washington, DC.

24. The National Foundation for the Treatment of Pain, "Perspectives in Intractable Pain Management," September 1, 2001, www.paincare.org/pain_management/perspectives/fear.html.

25. Letter from Dr. Benjamin R. Moore to Congressman Henry E. Brown, Jr., June 12, 2001.

26. The law enforcement agencies investigating Dr. Moore and other physicians in Woodward's clinic included the DEA Diversion Control Office in Columbia, the South Carolina Department of Health and Environmental Control (Bureau of Drug Control), the Hartsville Police Department, Darlington County Sheriff's Office, the South Carolina Department of of Health and Environmental Control, the Georgetown County Alcohol & Drug Abuse Commission, the Lancaster County Narcotics Office, and the U.S. Marshals Service Office in Florence, South Carolina.

27. Before 1984, the DEA could only revoke a physician's license to prescribe medication on three grounds: (1) if he falsified a prescription; (2) was convicted of a felony related to controlled substances; or (3) had his state medical license revoked or suspended. In 1984, Congress expanded the DEA's powers to criminalize physicians' narcotic pain prescriptions. The passage of the Dangerous Drug Diversion Control Act gave the DEA's Office of Diversion Control the discretionary power to revoke doctors' rights to prescribe medicine if it is not in the "public interest." The DEA can therefore ruin a physician's career without any hearing or charges being laid against him. It also means that thousands of patients who are being treated for acute pain are suddenly forced to withdraw from opiates without any medical supervision. Inevitably, it leads to increased hospital admissions due to severe symptoms, including seizures, deaths, and even suicide.

28. Dr. Farkas cited a large study done in the 1980s that found that only 4 patients became addicted out of 12,000 treated with opiates for pain. Robert Carlson, "DG Dispatch-AAEM: Risk of Addiction to Pain Relief is Small, Expert Says," *Doctor's Guide to Medical & Other News*, November 23, 2001, www.docguide.com/dg.nsf/DGNews/0EBCE61FF58E3C148525688C005E4A890.

29. According to Dr. Venkata Pulivarthi, M.D., who worked at Woodward's clinic with Dr. Moore, Ben Moore examined all of his patients. Moore routinely gave patients complete neurological exams, including deep tendon reflex tests. He recorded the tests in his patients' charts (Interview, January 5, 2002).

30. Drug Enforcement Administration, "Prehearing Statement on Behalf of the Government in the Matter of Benjamin R. Moore, D.O., August 1, 2001," 8–11.

31. Ibid., 24.

32. Ibid., 22–23.

33. United States Department of Justice, Drug Enforcement Administration, "Order to Show Cause Immediate Suspension of Registration of Benjamin R. Moore, D.O., June 8, 2001," 3–4.

34. Letter from Dr. Benjamin R. Moore to Congressman Henry E. Brown, Jr., June 12, 2001.

35. DEA, "Prehearing Statement on Behalf of the Government, August 1, 2001," 16.

36. Ibid.

37. Ibid., 21–22.

38. Ibid., 22.

CHAPTER 3

1. United States Department of Justice (DOJ), Deputy Attorney General Publications and Documents, Health Care Fraud Report Fiscal Year 1998, 2, http://www.usdoj.gov/dag/pubdoc/health98.htm.

2. Statement by Attorney General Janet Reno, March 6, 1997, http://www.usdoj.gov/opa/pr/1997/March97/095ag.htm.

3. Association of American Physicians and Surgeons, *AAPS News*, 56(9), (September 2000):1.

4. Sebastian Mallaby, "Drug Companies Cozy up to Doctors," *St. Petersburg Times* (May 4, 2002): 15A.

5. Melissa Kline Clements, Oklahoma City, as reported in *AAPS News*, 56(9) (September 2000): 4.

6. Department of Justice, News release, "Justice Recovers Record $1.6 Billion in Fraud Payments Highest Even for One Year Period," November 14, 2001, http://www.usdoj.gov/opa/pr/2001/November/01civ591.htm.

7. *The Psychiatric Times* (March 1989): 7.

8. Ibid.

9. The Department of Health and Human Services and the Department of Justice Health Care Fraud and Abuse Control Program, Annual Report for FY 2005, August 2006, 33–34.

10. Ibid., 39; The Department of Health and Human Services and the Department of Justice Health Care Fraud and Abuse Control Program, Annual Report for FY 2000, "Executive Summary," January 2001, 18–22.

11. *The Psychiatric Times* (March 1989): 5

12. See Paul Craig Roberts and Lawrence M. Stratton, *The Tyranny of Good Intentions* (Roseville, CA: FORUM, 2000). The authors discuss the concentration of power in the hands of prosecutors without effective checks and balances. Their "win-at-all-costs" attitude has led prosecutors to suppress evidence exonerating defendants, falsify evidence, use witnesses who are lying, mislead grand juries, and other misconduct.

13. Jane Orient points out that the government uses the fiction that senior citizens are the victims of Medicare fraud. In fact, the money paid into Social Security for health care is a miniscule part of the costs of health care for seniors. Health care costs are largely met by taxes from those in the workforce. Jane Orient, "Can 'Health Care Fraud' Be Ended?," *Medical Sentinel* (July/August 1998): 128.

14. *The Psychiatric Times* (October 1990): 29–30.

15. Jane Orient, M.D., "Statement to the Committee on the Judiciary Subcommittee on Commercial and Administrative Law," U.S. House of Representatives, May 7, 1998, http://216.109.125.130/search/cache?ei=UTF-8&p=D+McCarty+Tho.

16. *The Psychiatric Times* (October 1990): 29.

17. Roberts and Stratton, 169.

18. Howard Fishman, "New York Psychiatrist Acquitted of Medicaid Fraud Changes," *The Psychiatric Times* (December 1990): 41.

19. Donald Zerendow and Howard Fishman, "In the Interest of Justice: Abuses in Medifraud Investigations," *The Psychiatric Times* (September 1990): 27.

20. I am grateful to Nicholas Bartz, D.O., for this illustration, May 11, 2002.

21. *The Psychiatric Times* (September 1990): 27.

22. Ibid. (July 1990): 20.

23. Samuel Nigro, "Lawyers and Physicians' Notes," Unpublished manuscript, April 25, 1966.

24. *AAPS News* (December 2000): 4.

25. Genevieve Nowolinski, Office of Evaluation and Inspections, Office of Inspector General, HHS, "A Brief History of the HHS Office of Inspector General," June 2001, 9–10.

26. *The Psychiatric Times* (October 1990): 30.

27. Ibid. (June/August 1989): 11.

28. Ibid. (June/July 1990): 20–21.

29. Ibid. (August 1992): 10.

30. Ibid. (September 1990): 26.

31. Ibid. (August/September 1990): 25.

32. Ibid. (November 1990): 33.

33. Ibid. (August 1992): 11.

34. Ibid. (July 1990): 21.

35. Ibid., 20.

36. Ibid. (March 1989): 7.

37. Ibid. (July 1990): 20.

38. Ibid. (June 1990): 17.

39. Ibid. (March 1989): 8.

40. Ibid. (September 1990): 27.

41. Ibid.

42. Ibid. (November 1990): 32.

43. Interview with the editors of *Medicare Compliance Alert*, July 13, 1998.

CHAPTER 4

1. James V. Smith, Jr., "How the Dr. Vargo Case Got Out of Hand," *Shelby Promoter* (April 26, 2001): 1A, 7A.

2. Ibid.

3. Thomas A. Withers, Frederick Kramer, and Christopher L. Varner, "The Tao of the Health Care Fraud Trial," *USA Bulletin*, 45(2) (April 1997): 29–35.

4. Ibid., 29, 35.

5. Ibid., 29.

6. Ibid., 31.

7. Ibid., 32.

8. Ibid., 34.

9. Ibid., 33.

10. Undated letter from John P. Highsmith, M.D., to Mike Cotter, attorney for Dr. Patsy Vargo.

11. When Walz was asked why he had made the call, he said that he was doing Vargo a favor by alerting her to the danger. Interview with Dr. Jon Walz, M.D., June 13, 2002.

12. Gary A. Pacey, Special Agent (DCIS) Seattle Resident Agency, *Report of Investigation*, March 21, 1995, B-1.

13. Report of interview by Gary A. Pacey for the Investigation of Dr. Patsy Vargo, April 5, 1995, *Report of Investigation*, B-6.

14. Interview with Dr. Patsy Vargo, June 17, 2002; Undated letter from Colonel Kenneth Rashid to Michael W. Cotter, Attorney at Law representing Dr. Patsy Vargo.

15. James V. Smith, Jr., "Flawed Prosecution Fasco Worthy of Vaudeville, Except It's Not Funny," *Shelby Promoter* (March 20, 2001): 1A, 5A.

16. Letter from Randal A. Stewart, Resident Agent in Charge, Seattle Resident Agency of DCIS, to Michael W. Cotter, Attorney at Law for Dr. Patsy Vargo, June 6, 1997.

17. As reported by Carol Bradley, "Medical Fraud or Government Vendetta?" *The Great Falls Tribune* (April 15, 2001): 4A.

18. Glenn D. Littenberg, M.D., FACP, report entitled "U.S. v. Vargo," January 14, 2001, 8.

19. Kent J. Moore, American Academy of Family Physicians, Letter to Dr. Vargo, July 3, 1997.

20. Letter from Terry Ryan, M.D., "To Whom It May Concern," September 3, 1997.

21. Anne Finger, "Why Are the Feds Hounding This FP," *Medical Economics* (July 23, 2001): 22.

22. AFAA Audit Review Record, 3/23/96-6/12/96 #012463-012468 Malmstrom Air Force Base, V3.

23. Finger, "Why Are the Feds Hounding This FP," 24.

24. AAFAA Audit Review Record, 4/18/96012464, V2.

25. Letter from John W. Osment, DAFC, MCSE, MCP+1, Chief Information Officer, Department of the Air Force, Headquarters 341st Space Wing (AFSPC) Memorandum for AFOSI, Detachment 806 From: 341MDSS/SGSBI, August,19 1999.

26. Letter from Glenn D. Littenberg, M.D., FACP, to Charles Mitchell, Hogan & Hartson, LLP, January 14, 2001.

27. United States District Court, *Eastern District of Wisconsin, USA v. Dr. Allan Belden*, Case No. 99-CR-54, Milwaukee, Wisconsin, vol. 1, August 2, 1999, 35.

28. United States District Court, *Eastern District of Wisconsin, USA v. Allan Dinwoddie Belden, Jr., Presentence Investigation Report*, November 16, 2000, 17.

29. Trial Transcript, vol. 5, August 6, 1999, 957.

30. Trial Transcript vol. 7, August 10, 1999, 1142.

31. United States District Court, *Eastern District of Wisconsin, USA v. Allan D. Belden*, "Decision and Order," Case No. 99-CR-54, August 29, 2000, 8.

32. United States District Court, *Eastern District of Wisconsin, USA v. Allan D. Belden*, Transcript of Trial, vol. 7, August 10, 1999, 1207.

CHAPTER 5

1. Dalton, "Eye Physician's Home, Offices Raided," *The San Diego Tribune* (April 28, 1992): B-3.

2. Complaint Composite Exhibit 1, 018098, 3.

3. Richard P. Kusserow, Inspector General, OIG of the Department of Health and Human Services, "Outpatient Surgery, Medical Necessity and Quality of Care," February 1991, ii.

4. Ibid., 0-2.

5. McClatchy News Service, "Doctor Overseers Stand Accused," *The San Diego Union-Tribune* (August 25, 1992).

6. Donna Grubb, "The Medical Board of California: A Controversial Past, a Confusing Present, a Brighter Future?" *California Physician* (March 1993).

7. California Medical Board Hearing, Direct Examination of Thomas G. Thomas, January 20, 1993, 1–3.

8. Grubb, 51.

9. Ibid., 46–47.

10. California Medical Board Hearing, Direct Examination of Thomas G. Thomas.

11. Declaration of Glen C. Duncan, January 7, 1997, at San Diego, California.

12. Deposition by Carmen Chavez, August 11, 1997, Chula Vista, California.

13. Superior Court of the State of California for the County of San Diego, *Margaret Christensen, Plaintiff v. Jeffrey Rutgard, M.D., Shirley Stephene v. Jeffrey Rutgard, M.D.*, No. 659006 and No. 665895, vol. II of the Deposition of George V. Butera, December 21, 1993, 116–224.

14. Letter from Gene E. Royce to Hon Kevin Midlam re Confidential Settlement Conference Statement, April 30, 1997–April 29, 1997.

15. Charles M. Sevilla, Appellant's Opening Brief, *United States v. Dr. Jeffrey Jay Rutgard*, United States Court of Appeals for the Ninth Circuit, Case No. 95-50309, April 17, 1996.

16. Declaration of Harold Diaz, Chula Vista, California, December 30, 1992.

17. Declaration of Armando Gabriana, San Diego, California, March 17, 1993. Declaration of Virginia Robinson, San Diego, California, December 17, 1992. Numerous patients reported being harassed and intimidated by medical board investigator Gerald O'Donnell and Tracy Hutchinson who wore "Police" windbreakers on their visits to patients' homes. Some of the patients who felt intimidated but refused to sign the MBC's complaint form included Willa B. Greene, Elizabeth Chapman and Edgar Chapman, Nelda Griffin, Clayton Lackman, Ethyl Moody, Doris Flinn, Lois Denmon, Mary McDowell, Marjorie Alexander, Orville L. Evans, Barbara Norcott, Loneta Pegues, Steven and Jo-Ann Olson-Thompson, Lou Stapf, Harley Jones, M.D., Robert Morrisey, and Lt. Kenrick Harris.

18. Task Force Hearing on Quality of Medical Review, Medical Board of California Action Report, April 1994, 3.

19. Declaration by Henry I. Baylis, M.D., to the Medical Board of California, October 1, 1992.

20. Declaration of Dr. E. Lee Rice, D.O., San Diego, California, May 11, 1993.

21. Testimony of Dr. John M. Corboy, M.D., to the California Medical Board, January 11, 1993.

22. Ibid.

23. Appellant's Opening Brief, U.S. Court of Appeals, April 17, 1996, 49.

24. Ibid., 55.

25. Ibid., 57.

26. Declaration of Fred Chavez, San Diego, California, December 13, 1996.

27. Appellant's Opening Brief, U.S. Court of Appeals for the Ninth Circuit, April 17, 1996, 93–94.

28. http://www.blowthewhistle.com/falseclaimsact/facts2.html.

29. Request from Mike Cesaro of OIG-Office of Investigations (HHS Headquarters) to Marty Kriebel of the regional Office of Audit Services (Region III-OIG), July 25, 1988. Through Freedom of Information Request (FOIA) in 1996, Monika Krizek Griffis, Dr. Krizek's lawyer and daughter obtained 100 of 196 available documents that the HHS was willing to release.

30. Testimony of George O. Krizek, M.D., and Blanka H. Krizek, Subcommittee on Commercial and Administrative Law, Committee on the Judiciary, U.S. House of Representatives, May 7, 1998, http://www.house.gov/judiciary/5403.htm.

31. Transcript of Status Call Before the Honorable Stanley Sporkin, United States District Judge, Docket No. CR 93-54, Washington, DC, April 14, 1994, 42–43.

32. Trial Transcript, April 6, 1994, 6–7.

33. Ibid., 7–8.

34. Ibid., 9–10.

35. United States District Court for the District of Columbia, *United States of America v. George O. Krizek and Blanka H. Krizek*, Civil Action No. 93-54:A-54-A-55, January 1995.

36. Carolyn Tuft, "Dentist Accused of Murder Plot Wants Trial After 3 Years in Jail," *St. Louis Post-Dispatch* (September 15, 2000): A12.

37. Letter from Barry A. Short to C. Thomas Sell, D.D.S., January 30, 1998.

38. United States District Court, Eastern District of Missouri, *Eastern Division, USA v. Charles T. Sell*, Statement by Jane Ann Alderman, January 21, 1998, Cause No. 4, 97CR290, January 26, 1998, Exhibit A.

39. United States District Court, Cause No. 4, 97CR290, January 26, 1998, 5–6.

40. Motion of Defendant Charles T. Sell, D.D.S., for Revocation of the Bond Revocation and Detention Order, U.S. District Court, Eastern District of Missouri, *Eastern Division, U.S. v. Dr. Charles Thomas Sell*, D.D.S., No. 4, 97CR0290, February 9, 1998, 3.

41. Transcript of the Bond Revocation Hearing, 1998, 62.

42. Ibid., 31.

43. Transcript, 50.

44. Carolyn Tuft, *St. Louis Post-Dispatch* (June 19, 2003): A4.

45. Transcript, September 29, 1999, 10.

46. Transcript, Hearing on Involuntary Psychiatric Treatment and Medication, September 29, 1999, 122–123.

47. U.S. District Court Hearing, September 9, 1999, 49.

48. U.S. District Court Eastern District of Missouri, Eastern Division, Government's Response to the Defendant's Motion to Compel Production of Materials, August 28, 2000.

Chapter 6

1. Health Care Financing Administration (HCFA), *Medicare Fraud & Abuse: A Practical Guide of Proactive Measures to Avoid Becoming a Victim*, 2nd ed. (Jacksonville, FL: First Coast Service Options, 1999), 21.

2. Jeff Testerman, "Clinics Inquiry Reveals Web of Medicare Fraud," *St. Petersburg Times* (September 26, 1999): 4B.

3. Ibid.

4. Ibid.

5. Jeff Testerman, "Nominee Picked for U.S. Attorney," *St. Petersburg Times* (February 3, 2001):2.

6. G. Gassman, Clearwater Clinical Labs, Inc., *Physician Client File*, July 16, 1998.

7. Jane Meinhardt, "8 Facing Medicare Kickback Charges,"*St. Petersburg Times* (June 24, 1999): 3B.

8. Robert Farley and Ed Quioco, *St. Petersburg Times* (December 24, 2001): 3–4.

9. Inspector General, Department of Defense, Defense Criminal Investigative Service, Orlando Resident Agency, Investigations 9810215C-26-Jan-98-200R-I8Y, interview of Vincent Gepp.

10. United States District Court, Middle District of Florida, Tampa Division, *USA v. Michael Spuza and Ira Harvey Liss*, Case No. 8:99-CR-226-T-26A, April 17, 2000, 129.

11. U.S. District Court, Middle District of Florida, Search Warrant for Clearwater Clinical Laboratory, Case Number 98-272, June 8, 1998, 9.

12. Ibid.,12.

13. Inspector General, Department of Defense, Defense Criminal Investigative Service, 9810215C, January 20, 1998.

14. *U.S. v. Levine*, 546 F. 2d 658, 663-5th Cir., 1977.

15. Each of the doctors was given a copy of a letter dated February 11, 1993, from Jeffrey Sauey claiming that the space rental agreements for draw stations met the government's legal requirements. They also received copies of a letter from attorney Leslie Conklin, dated September 22, 1995, affirming the legality of personal service contracts such as MROs and TROs for CCL.

16. "Safe Harbors" referrals are permitted in three specific circumstances. Doctors are allowed to rent space in their offices, rent medical equipment, and receive payments from outside companies for their services. To qualify for safe harbor exemption, physicians must sign written agreements for at least one year, and the payments must be based on "fair market value."

17. U.S. District Court, Middle District of Florida, Tampa Division, Case No. 8:00-CR-226-T-26(A), April 7, 2000, 72.

18. Ibid., 75, 80.

19. Ibid., 133.

20. Ibid., 135.

21. Ibid.

22. Ibid., 37–38.

23. Trial Transcript, April 19, 2000, 85–86.

24. Trial Transcript, April 17, 2000, 29, lines 7–11.

25. Trial Transcript, April 20, 2000, 25–26.

26. Robert Farley and Ed Quioco, 2, 6.

CHAPTER 7

1. Drug Enforcement Agency, "OxyContin Special," vol. 1, 2001, 3, 9; Asa Hutchinson, Administrator, Drug Enforcement Administration, Congressional testimony before the House Committee on Appropriations Subcommittee for the Departments of Commerce, Justice, State, the Judiciary and Related Agencies, March 20, 2002; Domestic Strategic Intelligence Unit (NDAS), Office of Domestic Intelligence in coordination with Office of Diversion Control of the Drug Enforcement Administration, March 2002, 4.

2. Fred Schulte, "Deaths Mount as Doctors, Pharmacists and Patients Abuse the Medicaid System," *Sun Sentinel* (November 30, 2003): 1.

3. Personal communication from Dr. David Haddox, November 11, 2004; *Dow Jones Newswires*, "FDA Panel: OxyContin's Approval Shouldn't Be Limited," September 9, 2003. Four professional boards of medicine offer certification in pain management. As of November 2004, there were 5,869 physicians certified in pain medicine, not all of whom prescribe opiates for the treatment of chronic pain. The boards and the number of doctors certified are as follows: The American Board of

Anesthesiology (ABA)–3,127; American Board of Pain Medicine (ABPM)–1,768; American Board of Physical Medicine and Rehabilitation (ABPMR)–875; American Board of Psychiatry and Neurology (ABPN)–99. Personal communication from Kris Haskins, ABPM, November 11, 2004; Steve Glick, ABPN, November 17, 2004; Joseph McClintock, ABA, November 22, 2004; Donna Morris, ABPMR, November 17, 2004.

4. American Pain Foundation, "Talking Points on Pain," September 2004, http://www.painfoundation.org/print.asp?file=PCPA2003_Points.htm; Wisconsin Medical Society, "Guidelines for the Assessment and Management of Chronic Pain," *Wisconsin Medical Journal*, 103(3), 16.

5. Grier J. Wolfe, Klar N. Levein S.B., et al. "Symptoms and Suffering at the End of Life in Children with Cancer," *New England Journal of Medicine* 342 (2000): 326–333.

6. The American Pain Foundation, "Talking Points on Pain," http://www.painfoundation.org/print.asp?file=PCPA2003.htm; *AMNews* (September 23/30, 2002): 1.

7. David F. Musto, *The American Disease: Origins of Narcotic Control* (New York: Oxford University Press, 1999), 1–23; personal interview, January 23, 2004.

8. Dr. H. H Kane, "The Hypodermic Injection of Morphia, Its History, Advantages, and Dangers," as discussed by Edward M. Brecher and the editors of *Consumer Reports Magazine*, 1972, http://216.239.41/search?q=cache:jwt_JyEL.2AwJ:www.alb2c3com/drugs/opi003.htm.

9. Edward M. Brecher, *Licit and Illicit Drugs* (Boston: Little Brown & Co., 1973); Edward M. Brecher and the editors of *Consumer Reports Magazine*, "Opiate History, Nineteenth Century America," *Consumer Reports Magazine* (1972): 7–8.

10. Charles E. Terry and Mildred Pellens, *The Opium Program* (New York: Bureau of Social Hygiene, 1928).

11. Musto, "Race and the Drug War," *Drug Policy Alliance* (2004): 1–2.

12. Musto, *The American Disease*, 132–134.

13. Kurt Hohenstein, "Just What the Doctor Ordered: The Harrison Anti-Narcotic Act, the Supreme Court, and the Federal Regulation of Medical Practice, 1915–1919," *Journal of Supreme Court History*, 26, no. 3 (2001): 231–256.; David F. Musto, "Physicians' Attitudes toward Narcotics," in C.S. Hill, Jr., and W.S. Fields, eds., *Advances in Pain Research and Therapy*, vol. 11 (New York: Raven Press, 1989), 51–59.

14. The Harrison Narcotics Act (1914) Public Law No. 223, 63rd Congress (December 17, 1914), http://216.239.39.104/search?cache:fo_G4ccDpDEJ;www.erowid.org/psychoactives/law.

15. Harry G. Levine, "The Secret of Worldwide Drug Prohibition," *The Independent Review*, 7(2) (Fall 2002): 3; Eric Sterling, "Drug Policy Failure at Home," http://www.lightparty.com/foreignPolicy/DrugPolicyFailureATHome.html.

16. Hohenstein, "Just What the Doctor Ordered," 253; Musto, *The American Disease*, 181–182.

17. Musto, *The American Disease*, 121.

18. Rufus B. King, *The Drug Hang-Up: America's Fifty-Year Folly*, 2nd ed. (Springfield, IL: Charles C. Thomas, 1972); and "The Narcotics Bureau and the Harrison Act: Jailing the Healers and the Sick," *Yale Law Journal* (1953): 784–787.

19. Hohenstein, "Just What the Doctor Ordered," 245.

20. Edward Jay Epstein, *Agency of Fear: Opiates and Political Power in America* (New York: Verso, 1977), 104.

21. Musto, *The American Disease*, no. 6, 368; Hearings before the House Appropriation Committee, Treasury Department, Appropriation Bill 1930, November 23, 1928, 1st session, 473.

22. King, *The Drug Hang-Up: America's Fifty-Year Folly*, 786.

23. Musto, *The American Disease*, 59.

24. Edward M. Brecher and the editors of *Consumer Reports Magazine*, "The Pure-Food and Drug Act of 1906," *Consumer Reports Magazine* (1972): chapter 7, 1; Lawrence Kolb and A.G. Du Mez, *The Prevalence and Trend of Drug Addiction in the United States and Factors Influencing It*, Treasury Department, U.S. Public Health Service, Reprint No. 924 (Washington, DC: U.S. Government Printing Office, 1924), 14, Table 2.

25. Musto, *The American Disease*, 245–274, 268–269.

26. Ibid., 261–63; Kolb and Du Mez, "*Prevalence.*"

27. 21 USC 841 (b)(1)(a).

28. Timothy Lynch, "The Case Against Plea Bargaining," *Regulation*, 26(3) (Fall 2003): 24–27.

29. Bruce L. Benson, "The American Drug War: Anatomy of a Futile and Costly Police Action," The Independent Institute, Oakland, California, July 10, 2000, 8, http://64.233.161.104/search?q=cache:Jjb7FSGdxHOJ:independent.aristotle.net/publication.

30. Henry Hyde, *Forfeiting Our Property Rights: Is Your Property Safe from Seizure?* (Washington, DC: Cato Institute, 1995).

31. Prepared Remarks of Attorney General John Ashcroft, DEA/Drug Enforcement Rollout, March 19, 2002.

32. Josh White, "Pill Probe Focuses on N. Va Doctors," *Washington Post* (August 4, 2002): A01.

33. Federal Bureau of Prisons, *Quick Facts*, http://www.bop.gov/fact0598.html.

34. William B. Moffitt, President National Association of Criminal Defense Lawyers. Congressional testimony at hearing before the House Government Reform Subcommittee on Criminal Justice, Drug Policy and Human Resources on Drug Sentencing Policy, May 11, 2000.

35. Musto, *The American Disease*, 255; The Controlled Substances Act (CSA) is Title II of the Drug Abuse Prevention and Control Act of 1970. The Act initiated the "War on Drugs" and started a national campaign against illicit drugs and crime. The CSA gave the Bureau of Narcotics and Dangerous Drugs (BNDD) the authority to regulate legal prescription drugs. When the Drug Enforcement Agency was created in 1973, it acquired the BNDD's authority.

36. *United States v. Moore*, 423 U.S. 122, 124 (1975).

37. The Controlled Substances Act created five schedules of categories of drugs based upon their approved medical use and the potential to addict patients. Schedule I drugs, such as heroin and marijuana, have no approved medical use and were said to have a high potential for addiction. They are authorized for medical research only. Schedule II drugs are narcotics and nonnarcotics such as cocaine, methadone, Oxycodone, and OxyContin. They also include nonnarcotic drugs such as amphetamines and barbiturates that are approved for medical use but have the highest addictive

potential. Schedules II, IV, and V include drugs such as narcotics combined with non-narcotic drugs such as codeine and aspirin and caffeine and mild depressants and tranquilizers that have a low risk of addiction.

38. DEA Mission Statement, Drug Enforcement Administration, www.dea.gov/agency/mission.htm.

39. GAO/GGD-99-108, "Drug Control, DEA's Strategies and Operations in the 1990s" (Washington, DC: United States General Accounting Office, July 1999), 7, 61, 72–73, 78.

40. Department of Justice, "Status of Achieving Key Outcomes and Addressing Major Management Challenges," June 2001.

41. "Review of the Drug Enforcement Administration's (DEA) Control of the Diversion of Controlled Pharmaceuticals," The Drug Enforcement Administration, September 2002, http://www.usdoj.gov/oig/inspection/DEA/0210/Memo.htm.

42. U.S. Department of Justice, Drug Enforcement Administration, "Action Plan to Prevent the Diversion and Abuse of OxyContin," 2001; U.S. Department of Justice, Drug Enforcement Administration, "DEA-Industry Communicator: OxyContin Special," vol. 1. http://www.deadiversion.usdoj.gov/drugs_concern/oxycodone/abuse_oxy.htm.

43. Josh White and Marc Kaufman, "U.S. Compares Va. Pain Doctor to 'Crack Dealer,'" *Washington Post* (September 30, 2003):B03.

44. Statement of Asa Hutchinson, Administrator, Drug Enforcement Administration before the United States Senate Caucus on International Narcotics Control, Executive Summary, April 11, 2002, www.dea.gov/pubs/cngrtest/ct041102p.html.

45. Ibid., 1, 3–4.

46. U.S. Department of Justice, Drug Enforcement Administration, Diversion Control Program, "Summary of Medical Examiner Reports on Oxycodone-Related Deaths," May 16, 2002, www.deadiversion.usdoj.gov/drugs_concern/oxycodone/oxycotin7.htm.

47. Ibid., 4.

48. Ibid., 1.

49. "Oxycodone Involvement in Drug Abuse Deaths: A DAWN-Based Classification Scheme Applied to an Oxycodone Postmortem Database Containing Over 1000 Cases," *Journal of Analytical Toxicology*, 27(2) (March 2003):57–67.

50. DEA, "Summary of Medical Examiner Reports on Oxycodone-Related Deaths," 1.

51. Ibid., 4.

52. Mike Gray, *Drug Crazy* (New York: Routledge, 1988); see also Edward Jay Epstein, *Agency of Fear: Opiates and Political Power in America* (New York: Verso, 1990).

53. "Cocaine and Crack," National Drug Intelligence Center's National Drug Threat Assessment 2003, January 2003, http://www.usdoj.gov/ndic/pubs3/3300/cocaine.htm.

54. Tom Morganthau, "Crack and Crime," *Newsweek* (June 16, 1986):16.

55. Asa Hutchinson, Statement Before the House Committee on Appropriations, Subcommittee on Commerce, Justice, State, and Judiciary, December 11, 2001, 1; Hutchinson, April 11, 2002, 1.

56. Donna Gold, "A Prescription for Crime: A Bust of 2 Painkillers Blamed for Rise in Violence in Maine's Poorest County," *The Boston Globe* (May 21, 2000): D22.

57. Timothy Roche, "The Potent Perils of a Miracle Drug: OxyContin Is a Leading Treatment for Chronic Pain, but Officials Fear It May Succeed Crack Cocaine on the Street," *Time Magazine*, 157 (January 8, 2001):47.

58. Gary Cohen, "The Poor Man's Heroin," *U.S. News & World Report* (February 12, 2001):27.

59. Francis Clines and Barry Meier, *The New York Times* (February 9, 2001):A21.

60. Doris Bloodsworth, "OxyContin Under Fire," *Orlando Sentinel* (five part series) (October 19–23, 2003); Doris Bloodsworth, "Pain Pill Leaves Death Trail: A Nine-Month Investigation Raises Many Questions about Purdue Pharma's Powerful Drug OxyContin," *Orlando Sentinel* (October 19, 2003).

61. Manning Pynn, "A High Premium on Truth; A Lifelong Dread Realized," *Orlando Sentinel* (October 27, 2003); Kay R. Daly, "Painful Bias," *GOPUSA* (November 12, 2004):1.

62. Dan Tracy and Jim Leusner, "Orlando Sentinel Finishes Report about OxyContin Articles," *Sun Herald* (February 21, 2004):2, www.sunherald.com/mld/sunherald/news/nation/8010419.htm?template=contentMo; Doris Bloodsworth, "FDA Urged to Get Tougher on OxyContin Maker," *The Orlando Sentinel* (November 19, 2003):3, www.yourlawyer.com/practice/printnews.htm?story_id=7103.

63. "Congress Tackles OxyContin: Legislators' 1st Hearing Will Be in Orlando in February," *Orlando Sentinel* (December 5, 2003):2.

64. Doris Bloodsworth, "Crowd Protests Drug Maker: Dozens Who Had Lost Relatives and Friends to OxyContin Overdoses Braved the Rain Outside an Orlando Resort to Rally Against Manufacturer Purdue Pharma," *Orlando Sentinel* (November 20, 2003):3.

65. Ibid.

66. James R. McDonough, Testimony of James R. McDonough Before the Government Reform Committee, Subcommittee on Criminal Justice, Drug Policy and Human Resources, February 9, 2004.

67. United States General Accounting Office, "OxyContin Abuse and Diverson and Efforts to Address the Problem," GAO-04-110, December 2003,10.

68. Howard Kurtz, "After OxyContin Series: A Delayed Reaction," *Washington Post* (February 16, 2004):C01.

69. Dan Tracy and Jim Leusner, "Orlando Sentinel Finishes Report about OxyContin Articles," *Sun Herald* (February 21, 2004):1.

70. Florida Department of Law Enforcement, "2001 Report of Drugs Identified in Deceased Persons by Florida Medical Examiners," April 2001, 11; "2002 Report of Drugs Identified in Deceased Persons by Florida Medical Examiners," June 2002, 6.

71. The state medical examiners collected data on the following drugs: ethyl alcohol, benzodiazepine, cannabinoids, cocaine, GHB, heroin, hydrocodone, oxycodone, ketamine, methadone, methylated amphetyamines, nitrous oxide, phencyclidine (PCP), and rohypnol. 2002 Report on Drugs, i.

72. State medical examiners' 2001, Report on Drugs, 12; 2002 Report on Drugs, 7.

73. Orlando Business Journal, "Orlando Sentinel Reporter Resigns, Two Editors Reassigned in OxyContin Story Fallout," *Orlando Business Journal* (February 27, 2004):1; Trevor Butterworth, "The Great OxyContin Scare," *AlterNet: DrugReporter* (August 30, 2004):1, www.alternet.org/drugreporter/19707/.

74. Christy McKerney, "Doctor Charged with Murder Again," *Sun-Sentinel* (March 3, 2004):1.

75. Marc Kaufman, "DEA Withdraws Its Support of Guidelines on Painkillers," *Washington Post* (October 21, 2004):A03.

76. Thomas W. Raffanello, Statement of Thomas W. Raffanello, Special Agent in Charge, Miami Division, U.S. Drug Enforcement Administration before the U.S. House of Representatives Committee on Government Reform, Subcommittee on Criminal Justice, Drug Policy and Human Resources, February 9, 2004, 4.

77. Asa Hutchinson, "Statement before the U.S. Senate Caucus on International Narcotics Control," Executive Summary April 11, 2002, 5–8, www.dea.gov/pubs/cngrtest/ct041102p.html.

78. Appendix, Budget of the United States Government, Fiscal Year 1999, 606–609; DOCID, 1999-app-jus-7.

79. Hutchinson, "Statement before the U.S. Senate Caucus on International Narcotics Control," 7.

80. Rogelio E. Guevara, Statement of Rogelio E. Guevara, Chief of Operations, DEA before House Judiciary Committee, Subcommittee on Crime, Terrorism, and Homeland Security, May 6, 2003, 5, www.usdoj.gov/dea/pubs/cngrtest/ct050603p.htm.

81. DEA, "Drug Intelligence Brief": OxyContin, Pharmaceutical Diversion, March 2002, 5, www.usdoj.gov/dea/pubs/intel/02017/02017p.html.

82. Joe Burchell, Michael Marizco, and Enric Volante, "Hospital's Drug Theft Estimates Spiraling," *Arizona Daily Star* (June 24, 2004).

83. Associated Press, "Pill Thefts Alter the Look of Rural Drugstores," *The New York Times* (July 6, 2004).

84. Scott J. Orr, "Of Six Bogus Requests for Drugs over the Internet, Only One Was Denied," *The Star-Ledger* (November 30, 2003).

85. 21 USC Sec. 853 01/22/02, 1–2, www.usdoj.gov/dea/pubs/csa/853.htm.

86. DEA, News from DEA, Domestic Field Divisions, "Asset Forfeiture Benefits Local Police Departments," *Atlanta News Releases* (March 25, 2003).

87. U.S. Department of Justice, Office of Inspector General, Audit Division, "Assets Forfeiture Fund and Seized Asset Deposit Fund Annual Financial Statement Fiscal Year 2002," Report 03-20, June 2003, 1.

88. The National Association of Drug Diversion Investigators (NADDI) was founded in 1987, for the purpose of investigating and prosecuting pharmaceutical drug diversion. There are about 2,400 members of NADDI representing local and state and police departments, DEA agents, insurance investigators, drug companies and pharmacies loss prevention departments, and state medical board and pharmacy regulatory agents who investigate and prosecute the diversion of prescription drugs. It has 14 state chapters in Alabama, California, the Carolinas, Florida, Indiana, Kentucky, Maryland, New England, New York, Ohio, Pennsylvania, Tennessee, Texas, and Virginia. NADDI hosts training seminars for the purpose of coordinating methods of investigating and prosecuting drug diverters.

89. Dennis M. Luken, lecture on "Pharmaceutical Drug Diversion Schemes," National Association of Drug Diversion Investigators Training Conference, July 24, 2003.

90. John Burke, "Drug Diversion: The Scope of the Problem," *Le Technology Article* (November 26, 2004):5, www.naddi.org/states.asp.

91. Greg Aspinwall, Lecture on "Diversion of Non-Controlled Drugs," National Association of Drug Diversion Investigators Training Conference, July 24, 2003.

92. Ibid.

93. Luken, lecture, July 24, 2003.

94. DEA Diversion Control Program, "Rules-2003," *Federal Register*, 68(32) (February 18, 2003):5.

95. DEA Update, National Association of State Controlled Substance Authorities, Myrtle Beach, South Carolina, October 2002, 17–18.

96. DEA, Last Acts Partnership, Pain & Policy Studies Group, University of Wisconsin, "Prescription Pain Medications," 2004, 42–43.

97. DEA, "Briefs & Background, Drugs and Drug Abuse, Drug Description, Drug Classes," www.usdoj.gov/dea/concerndrug_classesp.html; DEA, "Historical Interviews, James McGivency," Tape No. 162, 2.

98. Laura Nagel, testifying for the DEA at a FDA hearing on the dangers of prescribing OxyContin, said, "In 60 percent of our criminal cases, the source of diversion was a physician or a pharmacist. The other 40 percent were drug thefts, doctor shoppers." Department of Health and Human Services, Food and Drug Administration, Center for Drug Evaluation and Research, "Anesthetic and Life Support Drugs," Advisory Committee, Wednesday, September 10, 2003, Bethesda, Maryland, 113; see also Special OxyContin Issue, vol. 1, 3.

99. Luken, lecture, July 24, 2003.

100. Gregg Wood, Health Care Fraud Investigator, United States Attorney's Office, Western District of Virginia, Healthcare Fraud Prevention & Funds Recover Summit, Washington, DC, June 21–23, 2004, 8–9.

101. DEA and Last Acts Partnership, Pain & Policy Studies Group, University of Wisconsin, August 2004; DEA, "Dispensing of Controlled Substances for the Treatment of Pain: Interim Policy Statement," posted on the DEA Web site, November 12, 2004, www.doctordeluca.com/Library/WOD/DEA-FAQ-InterimStatement111204.htm.

102. DEA, "Dispensing of Controlled Substances for the Treatment of Pain: Interim Policy Statement," November 12, 2004, 3.

103. Luken, lecture, July 24, 2003.

Chapter 8

1. Peter Franceschina, "Murder Trial Sparked Concern among Pain Specialists," *Sun-Sentinel* (Fort Lauderdale, FL) (May 20, 2005):1.

2. News-Journal Wire Services, "Panhandle Doctor's Oxycontin Conviction to Send Message," *News-Journal* (Daytona Beach, FL) (February 21, 2002).

3. Initial Brief of Appellant, First Judicial Circuit Court, Case No.1D02-1664, September 2003, W.C. McLain, 101.

4. Derek P. Ivnick, "Doctor, Free on Bond, to Be in Court August 7," *Pensacola News-Journal* (July 4, 2000):1A, 4A.

5. Ibid.

6. Dr. Graves was fired by Cracker Barrel restaurant in July 2001. James Graves explained on a Web site www.asappain.com that he was dismissed after Russ Edgar called the corporate headquarters of Cracker Barrel restaurant and "demanded that I be let go from my job as a bus boy and dishwasher because of the criminal charges filed against me." Dr. Graves claimed Edgar had previously gotten him fired from McDonalds by calling and informing them that they had a murderer working for them. On July 2, 2001, Graves filed an ethics complaint against Edgar with the Florida Bar Association. Russ Edgar denied he had called anyone, and FDLE Special Agent Dennis Norred testified during the trial that Cracker Barrel managers said that Graves was fired because of complaints from customers and coworkers. Monica Scandlen, *Pensacola News Journal* (September 7, 2001).

7. Derek Pivnick, *Pensacola News Journal* (November 5, 2005):A1, C4.

8. Affidavit for Search Warrant in the Circuit Court of the First Judicial Circuit of Florida, State of Florida, County of Santa Rosa before Circuit Judge, Kenneth B. Bell, April 1, 2000.

9. The Circuit Court of Santa Rosa County, Florida, *State of Florida v. James F. Graves*, Case No.:00-627-CFA, 00-422-CFA, Vol. 27, February 7, 2002, 5110.

10. Ibid., 5108.

11. Trial Transcript, vol. 20, January 31, 2002, 3632–3634, 3757–3758.

12. Monica Scandlen, "Doctors Who Deal, Not Heal, Targeted," PensacolaNewsJournal.com, February 26, 2002, 1A, 11A.

13. 2003 Tricare Healthcare Fraud Conference, "Tricare Top 50 OxyContin Prescribers in Florida, June 1996 to July 2000," 2003 Tricare Healthcare Fraud Conference, San Francisco, California, June 25–27.

14. Trial Transcript, vol. 21, February 1, 2002, 3888–3955.

15. Ibid., 3909.

16. Ibid., 3903.

17. Trial Transcript, vol. 21, January 31, 2002, 3826.

18. Trial Transcript, vol. 33, February 12, 2002, 6308–6413.

19. Ibid., 6403.

20. Trial Transcript, vol. 9, January 21, 2002, 1488.

21. Trial Transcript, vol. 28, February 7, 2002, 5216–5218 and vol. 33, February 12, 2002, 6289–6294, 6314–6329.

22. Trial Transcript, vol. 28, February 7, 2002, 5214–5223.

23. Trial Transcript, vol. 18, January 25, 2002, 3524–3527.

24. Trial Transcript, vol. 23, February 1, 2002, 4365.

25. Trial Transcript, vol. 31, February 12, 2002, 6059–6062 and vol. 34, February 12, 2002, 6483.

26. Trial Transcript, vol. 17, January 25, 2002, 3172.

27. Trial Transcript, vol. 17, January 25, 2002, 3176.

28. Affidavit for search warrant, April 1, 2000, 5.

29. Affidavit for search warrant, 5–6.

30. Monica Scandlen, PensacolaNewsJournal.com, February 26, 2002, A12.

31. Monica Scandlen, "Graves Guilty," Pensacola News Journal (February 20, 2002).

32. For example, Janet Johnson and James Gossett were not Dr. Graves' patients, and Donna Thompson and Theresa Kamper died after Dr. Graves' office closed and they were being treated by other doctors. James Longfellow saw Dr. Graves only once, and Samuel Jackson was dismissed after Graves learned that he was selling his drugs. Anne Carroll died from drugs purchased from a street dealer, Eddie Evans died after the removal of a lung due to a tumor, and James Campbell died after winning the lotto under suspicious circumstances following his marriage to a cocaine addict (personal communication from Dr. James Graves, December 29, 2005).

33. Carl T. Hall, *Chronicle Science Writer* (May 20, 2004).

34. Office of the Attorney General, Department of Justice, State of California, "Shasta County Physician, Two Pharmacy Operators Arrested for Felony Medi-Cal Fraud," February 19, 1999, Press Release, 99-021-a.

35. Kimberly Bolander, "Arraignments in Drug Case Are Delayed," *Redding Record Searchlight* (March 4, 1999).

36. "Doctor Likened to Drug Pusher, Prosecutor Says," *Sacramento Bee* (April 28, 1999):B3.

37. Wayne Wilson, "Shasta Trial Scheduled in Three Patient Deaths," *The Sacramento Bee* (January 2, 2002).

38. The term Siletz refers to approximately 30 small bands of American Indians totaling 15,000 that lived for thousands of years on the coast of northern California up to southern Washington. In 1850, there was a war between a tide of white prospectors looking for gold and the Siletz resisting this encroachment. The so-called Rogue River Wars lasted about six years with many of the remaining 6,000 Indians killed or dying of starvation and exposure. The survivors were forced by the U.S. Army to relocate to the Siletz Reservation. See Confederated Tribes of Siletz Indians, Siletz Community Health Clinic, 2004; James Mooney, "Siletz Indians," *The Catholic Encyclopedia,* vol. 13 (1912) and online edition (2003).

39. Indian Health Service, "Facts on Indian Health Disparities," Office of the Director/Public Affairs Staff, September 2002.

40. Centers for Disease Control and Prevention, "Morbidity and Mortality Weekly Report," vol. 52, no. 47 (Washington, DC: U.S. Government Printing Office, November 28, 2003), 1148–1152.

41. Personal communication from David Brushwood, R.Ph., J.D., University of Florida, October 31, 2004.

42. Skip Baker, "The Real Truth About the Case of Dr. Fisher in California," *The Unity Coalition,* November 24, 2001.

43. Jane Perkins, "Judicial Enforcement of Medi-Cal Laws and How It Is Evolving," *National Health Law Program,* April 23, 2004.

44. *Frank v. Kizer,* 213 Cal.App.3d 919,925,261 Cal Rptr. 882,297 (1989).

45. Perkins, "Judicial Enforcement of Medi-Cal Laws and How It Is Evolving."

46. Superior Court of California for the County of Shasta, People of the State of California, *Plaintiff v. Frank Fisher, et al., Defendant,* Case No. 99F1134, Proceedings May 18, 1999, 1450.

47. Ibid., 1370, 1390.

48. Ibid., 1393.

49. John Dodson, Affidavit and Statement of Probable Cause Experience of Affiant, February 1997, 4

50. Sam Stanton, "Murder Case Dissolved, but So Did Doctor's Life," *Sacramento Bee* (May 23, 2004).

51. Superior Court of California, 1999, 1402.

52. Ibid.

53. Ibid., 1380.

54. Superior Court of California, 1999, 1381.

55. Patrick S. Hallinan and Kenneth Wine, Defendant Frank Fisher's Notice of Motion and Motion to Dismiss under Penal Code 995, December 14, 1999, 19.

56. Ibid., 15.

57. Ibid., 9.

58. Ibid., 13. On February 2, 2005, six years after his medical clinic was raided, the last of four wrongful death suits against Dr. Fisher were dismissed. Two of the four civil plaintiffs were ordered to pay Fisher damages—$325.10 in one case and $1,022.54 in another one. Despite being completely exonerated, Frank Fisher was required by the California Medical Board to take a refresher course in general medicine and to have his narcotic prescriptions monitored by the board. See Maline Hazle, "Fisher's Ordeal Finally Is Over: Last of Four Death Suits Dismissed," *Record Searchlight,* Redding, California, February 2, 2005.

CHAPTER 9

1. Kenneth A. Gailliard, *The Sun News* (February 18, 2004):2, www.myrtlebeachonline,com/mld/sunnews/7978990.htm.

2. The case also involved the standard prosecution theory of criminality in DEA diversion cases and used criminals to testify that the doctors knew that they were addicts but supplied them drugs for money. This has been treated at length in Chapters 7 and 8. For example, prosecutors used the civil malpractice standard, "drugs were not 'medically necessary'" rather than the criminal standard "drugs were prescribed 'outside normal medical practice'" to convict the doctors. The case is also noteworthy insofar as the doctors were not linked to specific quantities of drugs but were assigned a share of the responsibility for the entire amount of drugs prescribed at the clinic.

3. District Court of the United States for the District of South Carolina, Florence Division, 2003. *United States of America v. David Michael Woodward*, Criminal No. 4:02-673, Plea Agreement, January 7, 2003.

4. Supra, Chapter 1.

5. Letter from B. Eliot Cole, M.D., Administrator, National Pain Data Bank and Pain Program Accreditation, Director, Continuing Medical Education, American Academy of Pain Management to Benjamin R. Moore, D.O., August 16, 2001.

6. United States of America, Ex Rel, *Deborah Bordeaux, M.D. v. David Michael Woodward, M.D.*, Comprehensive Care and Pain Management Center, Dr. David On Vandergriff, Myrtle Beach Medical Center, Pinnacle Health Care Systems, LLC., Grand Strand Imaging, Dr. Michael Jackson, Dr. Deborah Suterland, Dr. Michael Ross, Pamela Wagner, Dr. Vyeko Polic, Dr. Elizabeth Snoderly, Defendants August 7, 2001.

7. State Board of Medical Examiners of South Carolina, "Final Order" in the Matter of David Michael Woodward, M.D., Medical License #16747 (M-11-95) (M-42-95) Respondent, 1997, 12.

8. Undated private notes of Dr. Benjamin Moore.

9. State Board of Medical Examiners of South Carolina, Order on Remand, in the Matter of David Michael Woodward, M.D., Medical License #16747 (M-11-95)(M-42-95) Respondent, October, 21, 1998, 3.

10. State of South Carolina, County of Richland, *D. Michael Woodward, M.D., Appellant, v. South Carolina Department of Labor*, Licensing and Regulation, Division of Professional and Occupation Licensing Board of Medical Examiner, respondent. Court of Common Pleas, Fifth Judicial Circuit, Case No. 99-CP-40-1927, March 22, 2000, 10.

11. District Court of the United States for the District of South Carolina, Florence Division, Trial Transcript, January 30, 2003, 784.

12. Ibid., February 6, 2003, 1977.

13. Ibid., January 28, 2003, 307.

14. Dr. Gregory A. Walter, e-mails, February 28 and July 4, 2006.

15. Trial Transcript, January 30, 2003, 775.

16. Walter e-mail.

17. Traci Bridges, "Former Marion DSN Official Pleads Guilty in Federal Court," Channel 13 Morning News, December 21, 2001, 1.

18. On May 26, 2000, Dr. Moore talked to Mrs. Newton and Mickey McCully at the SC Board of Medical Examiners. Dr. Benjamin Moore's undated private notes.

19. Michael W. Woodward, "Pain Management Protocol," Comprehensive Care and Pain Management Center, Myrtle Beach, South Carolina, 1999.

20. State Board of Medical Examiners of South Carolina, *Guidelines for the Use of Controlled Substances for the Treatment of Pain*, February 1999.

21. Speech by Patricia M. Good entitled "The Drug Administration and Proposed Model Guidelines for the Use of Controlled Substances in Pain Management" before the Federation of State Medical Boards Symposium on Pain Management and State Regulatory Policy, Dallas, Texas, March 17, 1998.

22. United States Court of Appeals for the Fourth Circuit, Appeals from the United States District Court for the District of South Carolina, at Florence. C. Weston Houck, Senior District Judge (CR-02-673) Decided, December 1, 2005, 16, n. 11.

23. Trial Transcript, January 30, 2003, 821.

24. Ibid., 792.

25. Ibid.

26. Ibid., 823.

27. Ibid., 815.

28. Ibid., 1974.

29. Trial Transcript, February 5, 2003, 1869–1870.

30. Trial Transcript, January 30, 2003, 815.

31. Deborah Bordeaux, M.D., Letter Requesting a Change of Attorney Written August 16, 2002, to the Honorable C. Weston Houck, USDJ, District of South Carolina, Florence Division 401 W. Evans Street, Florence, SC 29501 and Honorable Thomas E. Rogers, III, USMJ, United States District Court, District of South Carolina, Florence Division 401 W. Evans Street, Florence, SC 29501. Case Number 4:02-673-05. Defendant Deborah Bordeaux, M.D., and Court Appointed Attorney R. Scott Joye.

32. On December 1, 2005, a three-judge panel of the Fourth Circuit Court of Appeals ruled that the three doctors were entitled to a new sentencing because of the U.S. Supreme Court's ruling in *U.S. v. Booker* earlier in the year that mandatory federal sentencing guidelines violated a defendant's Sixth Amendment right to a jury trial. Guidelines were now only advisory. On appeal, the sentences were reduced to two years for Alerre and Bordeaux and 2.5 years for Jackson.

INDEX

About the Author

RONALD T. LIBBY is Professor of Political Science and Senior Research Fellow at the Blue Cross and Blue Shield Florida Center for Ethics, Public Policy and the Professions at the University of North Florida. He is the author of five books and many articles including a widely discussed policy paper titled, "Treating Doctors as Drug Dealers," published by the Cato Institute.